Therapeutic Storytelling for Adolescents and Young Adults

Therapeutic Storytelling for Adolescents and Young Adults

Johanna Slivinske, MSW

Youngstown State University,
Youngstown, Ohio

Lee Slivinske, PhD

Youngstown State University,
Youngstown, Ohio

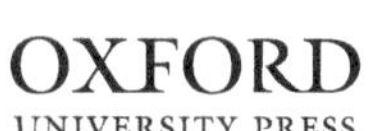

OXFORD
UNIVERSITY PRESS

Oxford University Press is a department of the University of Oxford.
It furthers the University's objective of excellence in research, scholarship,
and education by publishing worldwide.

Oxford New York
Auckland Cape Town Dar es Salaam Hong Kong Karachi
Kuala Lumpur Madrid Melbourne Mexico City Nairobi
New Delhi Shanghai Taipei Toronto

With offices in
Argentina Austria Brazil Chile Czech Republic France Greece
Guatemala Hungary Italy Japan Poland Portugal Singapore
South Korea Switzerland Thailand Turkey Ukraine Vietnam

Published in the United States of America by
Oxford University Press
198 Madison Avenue, New York, NY 10016

Library of Congress Cataloging-in-Publication Data
Therapeutic storytelling for adolescents and young adults / Johanna Slivinske, MSW, Youngstown
State University Adjunct Faculty, Department of Social Work Affiliated Faculty, Department of Women's Studies
Mental Health Therapist, PsyCare Inc., Lee Slivinske, PhD, Youngstown State University Professor Emeritus,
Department of Social Work.
pages cm
ISBN 978-0-19-933517-6 (pbk. : alk. paper) 1. Narrative therapy. 2. Child psychotherapy.
3. Family psychotherapy. I. Slivinske, Lee. II. Title.
RJ505.S75S646 2013
618.92'89165—dc23
2013023793

9 8 7 6 5 4 3 2 1
Printed in the United States of America
on acid-free paper

This book is dedicated to our talented daughter, Ashley Slivinske, from whom we continue to learn.

Contents

Foreword

Johanna is a lifelong friend and confidante with whom I have experienced over thirty years of friendship. Beginning in fifth or sixth grade, we have navigated the complicated, new emotions of adolescence and young adulthood together. We got into trouble in seventh grade science class (*Mad Magazine* does not qualify as scientific reading), played in the high school band, and talked about boys, among other things. Johanna's new work, *Therapeutic Storytelling for Adolescents and Young Adults*, picks up where *Storytelling and Other Activities for Children in Therapy* left off. Johanna and her coauthor Lee have had the insight to realize that not only is storytelling as therapy beneficial for children, but also that it can be continued with great success to help adolescents and young adults. Their book has delivered insight to many challenging moments of my early life and the life I share with my husband and three children.

Johanna and Lee have written yet another outstanding book on storytelling as therapy to express the complex feelings of adolescence and young adulthood that are unique to this stage of life. The topics are wide-ranging and geared to address the pressures, fears, doubts, and even joy that teens experience in our world today. Some topics may be familiar, such as the chapter "Parents." Oh, how I could have written a chapter on the wrongs my parents committed during my adolescence. They wouldn't let me do anything. All my friends would go to the mall, but I wasn't allowed to go. No one was going to invite me to do anything, since I was never allowed out of the house. Why were they so strict? Of course, looking back, my parents probably were on the stricter side, but I can appreciate why they were like that now that I am a parent. At the time, though, it was really rough. It would have been so helpful if my parents or I had had a resource to turn to for finding some sort of happy medium between my growing need for independence and my parents trying to protect me from the hurt they knew existed in the real world. As a mother with children transitioning between childhood and adolescence, I have found Johanna and Lee's advice invaluable.

While topics like this and others are familiar to those of us in the "older generation," Johanna and Lee have also included chapters in the book that address situations that are unique to today's adolescents and young adults, such as online exploitation, international violence, and issues of cultural and religious diversity. These topics are wide-ranging and geared to address the pressures, fears, doubts, and even joy that adolescents and young adults experience in our world today. The chapters offer a springboard for opening dialogue between adolescents and young adults and their parents, doctors, and counselors. Johanna and Lee's book is an important tool to help young people work through these tumultuous yet exciting years of growing up. It is more than a resource for professionals; it is a needed volume in the lives of all parents in the changing educational, technological, and political landscape.

Hester Doyle, PhD
Yale University, New Haven, CT

Preface

Take a moment to reflect on your own adolescence and young adulthood. What does it mean to you? Did you enjoy it? Did you despise it? It is a fanciful and joyous time for many, full of memories of carefree times, friendships, and romance. For others, it represents a time of despicable demons, unmet needs, and unfulfilled promises. Some may fit somewhere in the crack between happiness and depression. Others may still be trying to iron out the residual confusion from an identity not so firmly established.

As we recall the years of our adolescence and young adulthood, we are drawn to reflect and remember those who did not survive this precarious time. Some became lost to alcohol or drugs, others to suicide or homicide, others to victimization, yet others to the heartbreak of accidents, all too common during this time of life. We consider ourselves lucky. We are the survivors who have made it into middle age and older adulthood. We feel fortunate to be in this world, and we feel it a privilege to share what we have learned to help adolescents and young adults as they muddle through the quagmire of identity formation and intimate relationships.

This book has meaning for us on a variety of levels. We have both taught and counseled teens and young adults while they are in the midst of personal, academic, and professional development. Many of those with whom we work overcome seemingly insurmountable challenges on a day-to-day basis just to be able to survive. Their grit and resilience in life inspires and motivates us to write. We write to help others, and we write about life. Although the stories in this book are fictional, they are based on common themes that occur in many lives. They reflect the joyous, the inconsolable, and the monstrous moments from the collective consciousness of the lives of everyone, everywhere. They also reflect the resourcefulness and inner strengths needed to succeed and overcome life's challenges as experienced by adolescents and young adults.

We call on you, as clinicians and other helping professionals, to continue to fight the good fight in the quest to guide the younger generation toward a brighter tomorrow. By helping adolescents and young adults lay a solid foundation for their lives you, in turn, help us all. Thank you! What you do does matter.

Johanna Slivinske
Lee Slivinske

Acknowledgments

We would like to acknowledge the girl who spoke out at the meeting, the young man who ran for help, and all of you out there who are like them. You cared and were brave enough to do what you needed to do, and for that, we thank you. You make a difference in the lives of others, and that makes a difference to us.

We would like to thank our friends, family, and colleagues from Youngstown State University and PsyCare who encouraged us while we wrote this book. For supporting us in our journey, we extend special acknowledgment to our colleagues: Dr. Joseph L. Mosca, Mr. Joseph Mistovich, and Mr. Loren D'Amore. In addition, we thank Mr. Carl Leet for the exceptional photographs he contributed to the book. We recognize the staff at Maag Library at Youngstown State University who so graciously assisted us in obtaining needed materials for this book. For recognizing the value of our narrative work, we are grateful to our editor, Mr. Dana Bliss, our editorial assistant, Brianna Marron, our production editor, Reny Edwin Joseph, our copy editor, Suzanne Copenhagen and Oxford University Press. For continuing to teach us about life, we thank our students and clients. We are most grateful to our daughter, Ashley Slivinske, for whom this book is dedicated, for permission to use her story, "Roller Coaster." In memoriam, we thank our parents who continued to love and support us as teens and young adults.

Johanna Slivinske
Lee Slivinske

Introduction

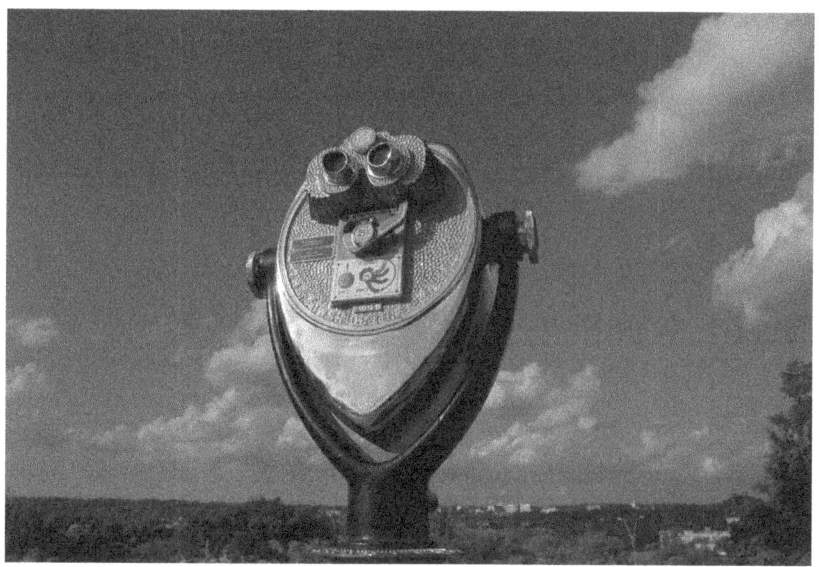

Everyone has a story to tell, and everyone deserves to have his or her story told. The war veteran who has recently returned to civilian life, the teenage girl who was sexually assaulted on her way home from practice, the young adult who cannot find a well-paying job—this book was written to help them to tell their stories and to help them to heal their emotional wounds and recover from traumatic events. That is what this book is about. We want adolescents and young adults to tell their stories. We want them to have a voice, to share their experiences and emotions, and to create their futures through their stories. Storytelling is an activity that comes naturally to many people, and it has been used as a form of artistic expression across cultures, landscapes, and points in time. The healing power of the narrative and its intertwining with the expressive arts continues to propel people to tell, write, and produce different ways to tell their stories, including the use of the oral tradition, written narrative, and artistic expression.

This book provides therapists with the knowledge, insight, and tools needed to assist adolescents and young adults overcome a variety of developmental, personal, and social issues by using a narrative type approach to storytelling and other therapeutic activities. It also helps them find the resources and strengths needed to succeed in their dynamic, ever changing environment. Stories and activities relating to issues commonly faced by these youth include relevant practice issues such as dating violence, substance abuse, illness and disability, sexuality, trauma, school issues, relationships, eating issues, death, community violence and gangs, emotions, relationships, cultural and religious issues, job loss and poverty, and social adjustment and peer acceptance, to name a few. Stories can be personalized by the therapists to meet the individual needs of their clients.

The activity questions and exercises that follow the stories reflect four levels of self-disclosure. Level-one activity questions are the least threatening and require the least amount of self-disclosure and insight, as they are about the life situations of others. Level-two questions require slightly more self-disclosure and generally are about people the client knows or knows of. This enables clients to discuss emotionally challenging material through a less threatening medium than directly addressing issues within themselves. Level-three questions involve higher levels of disclosure and are directed at situations in the life of the youth. Finally, level-four requires the highest level of intensity and disclosure, that of asking the youth to directly write his or her own story from beginning to end.

All chapters contain additional resources for those who desire to delve deeper into the matter contained therein. Here is a summary of chapter content. Thought-provoking stories and related questions are included in each of the special topic chapters numbered 6 through 24.

Chapter 1, Instructional Guidelines and Strategies, introduces the concepts of storytelling, narrative, writing, phototherapy, and other therapeutic artistic endeavors. It explains that the book contains overview chapters regarding its conceptual framework and supporting research and evidence, principles and processes of storytelling, developmental issues of adolescence and young adulthood, and the strengths-based approach to storytelling. It further explains that it is arranged by key practice areas, easy to locate and access, that contain sample stories and suggested questions to be answered by clients. It also offers suggestions for customizing the stories to meet the highly individualized needs of clients. The chapter introduces the Gradual Self-Disclosure Storytelling Technique, which comprises four graduated levels of questions and client self-disclosure. Finally, it defines and discusses various forms and uses of visual artistic expression in therapeutic settings.

Chapter 2, Conceptual Framework and Evidence-Based Practice, describes the overall conceptual framework used in this book, which includes the mutual storytelling techniques of Gardner, the narrative therapy of White and Epston, and the strengths-based perspective of Saleebey. Gardner proposes that therapists, upon hearing clients' stories, should select important themes, use the same characters, and create stories that have more positive outcomes. White and Epston assert that after stories are told, therapists should assist clients deconstruct them by assigning meaning and guiding clients in the externalization of their problems. Stories are then retold to develop a more positive direction. Saleebey proposes that therapists and clients together should find meaning in the stories and attempt to promote clients' gifts, assets, and strengths. After noting the similarities and differences among the various frameworks, the chapter reviews a number of qualitative and quantitative research studies that offer evidence for the effectiveness of storytelling and related narrative techniques.

Chapter 3, Principles and Processes of Storytelling with Teens and Young Adults, discusses the history, principles, and processes of storytelling. Throughout history, stories have been used to pass on knowledge and wisdom, cultural beliefs, and values and to instruct people on how to act in a variety of life's situations. Storytelling has been found to be an effective method for reaching adolescents and young adults as they can often relate to and identify with the characters in the stories and discuss with therapists what the characters may be thinking and what they should be doing in their respective situations. Relating to and discussing the problems of others tends to be less threatening than discussing their own personal issues directly. When ready, adolescents and young adults can use stories to self-disclose and retell the stories to gain insight into themselves and others and to develop more positive solutions to their problems.

Chapter 4, Developmental Issues of Adolescence and Young Adulthood, examines developmental issues facing adolescents and young adults. Youth encounter major physiological and hormonal changes, including the onset of secondary sex characteristics such as growth of facial and pubic hair, breast development, menarche, deepening of voice, and the like. Some of their reactions to these major bodily changes may include increased moodiness, feelings of sadness or sullenness, and aggressive or acting-out behaviors. During this life stage youth are struggling to formulate their own identities. In Western cultures, adolescents and young adults are expected to break away from parental control and experiment with various life roles and value systems. As a result of this search for independence, parental conflicts often result. Both family and peer relationships are important. Finally, the chapter reviews Erikson's developmental stages of identity versus role confusion and intimacy versus isolation, including important issues surrounding each.

Chapter 5, The Strengths Approach to Storytelling with Adolescents and Young Adults, points out that therapists should use the strengths-based approach in storytelling to assist teens and young adults identify their inner gifts, family supports, friendships (past and present), abilities, desire for change, and community-based opportunities and assets. Cultural beliefs, spirituality, and religious values and beliefs can also be built on to solidify a foundation for growth and healthy development. These strengths may be used to construct a mutually developed action plan for self-discovery and positive change.

They also may be used to help clients cope more effectively with past, present, and future issues in their lives. Past problems and dysfunctions should not be minimized and they should be dealt with, but they do not necessarily need to be the sole focus of intervention. The chapter provides a number of suggested strengths-based questions and statements. Finally, the chapter introduces our PLAN method of intervention. The PLAN method of intervention provides concrete steps and actions that can be taken to formulate goals, action plans, and build upon strengths. It involves positive action, looking to the future, activating strengths, and never giving up on yourself.

Chapter 6, Social Adjustment and Peer Acceptance, discusses the importance of adolescents and young adults adjusting to their social roles and being accepted by their peers. During this time of life some teens may struggle with trying to fit into a peer group and may need assistance learning social skills. Having positive, healthy relationships can boost teens' self-esteem and self-concept; not having such relationships can lead to pain, frustration, isolation, and loneliness. Negative peer influences that lead to destructive activities and behaviors must also be dealt with during this challenging and confusing period of life. The chapter offers practitioners suggestions for helping adolescents and young adults improve their self-esteem, social skills, and valuable relationships, as well as practice positive self-care.

Chapter 7, Sexuality, addresses the issues surrounding becoming sexually active and its consequences. During this life stage, youth are experiencing hormonal changes that result in increased libido. It is a time of curiosity and exploration regarding relationships and sexuality. This period in the life of teens and young adults may be fascinating and exciting and simultaneously bewildering and confusing. Many may experiment with different aspects of intimacy and sexuality on their road to adulthood. The chapter reviews the challenges regarding relationships and sexuality, discusses high-risk behaviors and the role of social media on sexuality, talks about the duties and responsibilities of having children, and shares tips to help young people who are struggling with their sexuality.

Chapter 8, Abuse, Sexual Assault, and Exploitation, addresses the level of incidence and consequences of abuse, sexual assault, and exploitation of adolescents and young adults. Some possible deleterious outcomes of these negative experiences include substance abuse, depression, anxiety, post-traumatic stress reactions, lack of trust in relationships, lack of control, anger issues, delinquency, and the like. Those who were abused, assaulted, or exploited by someone of the same sex may experience concerns or confusion regarding their sexual identity. Therapists who are assisting victims of abuse or assault must provide sincere emotional support and assure victims that they are not at fault. The chapter offers some solution-focused methods that concentrate on strengths-oriented questioning to promote growth.

Chapter 9, Parents, discusses the importance of parental relationships in the adolescent and young adult stages of development. As adolescents break away from their parents to establish their own unique identities, conflicts with parents often arise. These conflicts may also extend well into young adulthood, since many youth are now remaining at home for longer periods. This situation may contribute to increased friction in the home and the potential for confusion of roles and responsibilities regarding issues such as household chores, finances, and privacy, to name a few. The chapter also discusses problems and issues associated with divorce and incarceration and offers suggestions for parents and adolescents about dealing with relationship changes or conflicts.

Chapter 10, Relationships, explains that relationship issues and forming individual identities are key concepts central to developing into healthy teenagers and young adults. The importance of having positive and satisfying relationships during adolescence and young adulthood cannot be overstated, as such relationships have been found to be associated with increased emotional, cognitive, and social abilities. Individuals who experience them are more likely to become independent, productive adults. On the other hand, poor parental and peer relationships have been found to be associated with having fewer friends, higher levels of depression and drug use, and lower grade point averages. Therefore, therapists must always delve into the nature, extent, and types of relationships that adolescents and young adults are experiencing. The chapter offers tips for encouraging positive relationship skills in adolescence.

Chapter 11, Eating Issues, states that adolescents and young adults are at risk for encountering physical and mental health problems surrounding weight, diet, and nutritional issues. Negative health consequences may occur as a result of overeating, binge eating, dieting excessively, binging and vomiting, or abusing laxatives. Besides the physical problems such as diabetes, arthritis, heart disease, stroke, and cancers associated with obesity, a variety of social problems may occur as well. At any age, a social stigma may be attached to being overweight. This can be particularly difficult to handle during adolescence, when peer acceptance and the further development of self-concepts are simultaneously occurring. The chapter discusses problems associated with anorexia and bulimia, as well as providing suggestions to help teens with problems resulting in binge or addictive eating.

Chapter 12, Emotions, addresses how transitional life events in the lives of adolescents and young adults may trigger feelings of sadness, anger, and stress, including temporary or long-term feelings of depression and anxiety. All of these issues may also play a part in lowering an individual's self-concept. When faced with stressful or challenging life circumstances, individuals sometimes tend to maladaptively handle these events through either the internalization or externalization of their emotions. Those who internalize their emotions typically blame themselves and feel anxious and depressed. Those who externalize their emotions usually blame others and engage in acting-out behaviors such as punching walls, driving too fast, and being aggressive toward others. Major life events that trigger problems are listed as well as suggestions for positive ways of coping.

Chapter 13, Dating Violence, points out the negative consequences of dating violence for adolescents and young adults. At a minimum dating violence can be damaging to an individual's self-esteem. It also can result in serious injury or death. The chapter lists the various forms of dating violence, such as verbal, emotional, physical, and sexual and describes signs that may indicate that teens or young adults are in abusive relationships. Examples include being controlled or being controlling, extreme feelings of jealousy on the part of the violent partner, submissive behavior on the part of the nonabusive partner, and changes in behavior. The chapter offers general suggestions for practitioners to help ameliorate these situations.

Chapter 14, Substance Abuse, deals with the reality that many adolescents and young adults experiment with using drugs and alcohol. Some will become addicted to substances; addiction impacts their current and future relationships, academic performance, career aspirations, and other important areas of life functioning. The chapter examines factors that contribute to addictive behavior, such as peer pressure, imitation of parental drinking, easy access to alcohol or drugs, lack of supervision, and negative life events, as well as gender and racial differences in addictive behavior.

Chapter 15, Trauma, explains that during adolescence and young adulthood many individuals often engage in high-risk behaviors. It discusses the consequences of automobile and motorcycle accidents, shootings, and accidents or injuries from falls or stunts as well as the major causes of brain injury and death. It also addresses trauma from natural disasters such as earthquakes, hurricanes, tsunamis, floods, tornadoes, and fires as well as international events such as war. Finally it describes the signs and symptoms of post-traumatic stress.

Chapter 16, Military Issues and International Violence, address teenagers and young adults who may have family members, friends, boyfriends, girlfriends, or spouses who serve or have served in the military. Young adults themselves also may have been deployed. Military service impacts the relationships of everyone. The emotions experienced can range from feeling proud for serving one's country to feeling anger, disappointment, and sadness for missing significant life events at home. There is the constant worry about a safe and healthy return and the fear of death. Those who served may return with physical or mental challenges associated with their experiences or injuries endured while serving in the military. The chapter also deals with the feelings of those left behind and reactions to the deployment of a parent.

Chapter 17, Death, addresses how adolescents and young adults respond to death and dying. Responses to death become more complicated when additional developmental crises are present, such as trying to solidify one's own identity or attempting to nurture an intimate relationship. If multiple losses occur very close together, as they do for some, bereavement overload may occur, which in turn may cause the grieving process to shut down or manifest itself in various somatic symptoms. The chapter discusses the grieving process in relation to temperament, personality, culture, religion, gender, developmental stage, and so forth. It also explores additional influences surrounding this process, and it describes the five stages of death and dying from the work of Elisabeth Kübler-Ross.

Chapter 18, Strengths, emphasizes the strengths perspective, which uses ideas from positive psychology to assist therapists in fostering clients' human potential, fulfillment, happiness, and resilience. It serves as an adaptable and malleable framework that can be applied to numerous and varied life circumstances, including the assessment of systems of all sizes, such as individuals, families, groups, organizations, and communities. In addition, it respects and builds upon aspects of culture and diversity. The pain and hardship in individuals' lives must be valued and expressed, prior to moving forward to identify personal strengths. The chapter lists strengths for therapists to search for, as well as questions suggested by strengths-based proponent Dennis Saleebey.

Chapter 19, Community Violence and Gangs, discusses how community violence and gangs affect many different cross sections of society. Shootings and stabbings involving drugs and gang violence are common in certain neighborhoods. They disproportionately occur in many urban areas where crime, poverty, and drug abuse are prevalent. However, gun and other types of violence such as assaults, robberies, and rapes can and do occur in nearly every type of community, including suburban and rural neighborhoods. Individuals between the ages of 12 to 19 are two to three times more likely to be victims of the aforementioned crimes than adults in general.

Chapter 20, Independence, reviews the developmental processes of forming an identity and becoming independent. Tasks to be mastered to achieve independence include the ability to earn and manage money, shop for groceries and cook, maintain a clean living environment, and care for one's self and sometimes for others. The readiness to develop and use these skills will vary markedly from person to person based on maturity level and prior knowledge and skills. Problems may be encountered for those who may lack long-term financial, emotional, and social support or who have mental or physical disabilities. The chapter lists tips for how to become independent.

Chapter 21, Cultural and Religious Issues, examines how the culture in which adolescents and young adults are raised enables therapists to gain insight into their system of beliefs, values, and behavior. Understanding the cultural frameworks of clients enables practitioners to better meet their needs and to increase the effectiveness of treatment when adolescents and young adults are adjusting to the biological and psychological changes and increased social responsibilities associated with these life phases. Understanding the influence of religion also helps the therapist understand how to more effectively treat these individuals. The chapter discusses problems regarding bullying, sexual orientation, depression, and anxiety, among others, and provides strengths-based suggestions to aid therapists.

Chapter 22, Job Loss and Poverty, defines poverty as the extent to which a person lacks resources. Resources include clean water, food, clothing, housing, well-paying jobs or career opportunities, adequate social supports to assist with family functioning, educational opportunities, safe neighborhoods, recreational activities, and the like. The economic environment in which one grows and develops affects both current and future human development. Not being able to find gainful employment or being underemployed also hinders young adults from becoming independent and diminishes their chances for attaining educational and relationship goals, such as obtaining a degree or marriage. The chapter discusses the consequences of living in poverty and the factors that foster economic growth.

Chapter 23, Illness and Disability, discusses the difficulty of adapting to illness or disability of oneself, a friend, or family member. When illness or disability strikes, its ripples tend to be felt by everyone close to the person directly affected. Depending upon the type, quality, and characteristics of a mental or physical illness or challenge, these ripples may be small or large. The chapter offers suggestions for therapists who are assisting those with illness and disability. It lists and defines the Tuttles' seven phases of adjusting to blindness, which include physical or social trauma, shock and denial, mourning and withdrawal, succumbing and depression, reassessment and reaffirmation, coping and mobilization, and self-acceptance and self-esteem.

Chapter 24, School Issues, examines the positive and negative challenges encountered in school and college. Stress and anxiety regarding earning high marks, test-taking, or low grades and failure may contribute to feelings of academic pressure and tension. For those students predisposed to high anxiety, meditation, breathing exercises, and relaxation exercises may be practiced with the client in-session. These rehearsals may then be applied in the real test-taking environment. For students with poor study habits, review courses surrounding the particulars of how to study and ways to improve organization and efficiency may be of benefit.

The book concludes with Chapter 25, General Activities for All Practice Areas. The titles of the activities provided are: Where Am I? Activity, Relaxation Exercise Activity, Imagined Traits Relaxation Activity, My Story, Strengths Activity: The PLAN Method of Intervention, Activity: Positive Action Creates Positive Change, Strengths Activity: Look to the Future, Strengths Activity: My Plan Leads to My Future, Writing Activity, Thinking Outside the Box about Yourself, Strengths and Areas Needing Growth in Your Community Activity, Create a Video Game Activity, Steps I Can Take Activity, What are My Options?, Poem Activity, Steps I Can Take Activity, My Sexuality Activity, Personal Choices Activity, Coping Skills Activity, and Lifemap Activity.

Website, The companion website for this book contains color photographs for each chapter and related stories, activity sheets, and exercises that may be printed and used in therapeutic sessions. All of the color photographs can be used in phototherapy, while some are appropriate as points of focus for guided imagery. Additional resources and links to pertinent websites are also included for those who desire to explore each topic in greater detail and depth. Again, the stories may be personalized by therapists to meet their therapeutic goals and the individual needs of the adolescents and young adults in therapy. The activity sheets and exercises are user friendly and ready for immediate utilization.

Photographs, Again, the color photographs included on the website for each chapter relate to the content of each chapter and were purposefully selected with the intent of being used in phototherapy. Identical black and white photographs are included in the book. Copies of these photographs can be made and shown to clients with the intent of helping them delve deeper into their thoughts, feelings, emotions, and narratives. Some photographs are included to promote relaxation and can be utilized as tools for guided imagery, while others are more thought-provoking and are designed as a springboard to facilitate discussion, writing, and artistic expression. For example, a photograph of binoculars overlooking a panoramic view of a blue sky with white clouds is included in the Introduction. It was selected as to us it represents looking at a calming, beautiful horizon. Perhaps with a creative imagination or with the aid of a therapist clients might be able to figuratively or symbolically look into their futures to imagine what lies ahead in their lives. Another example is the photograph of a car that is provided for Chapter 6, Social Adjustment and Peer Acceptance. It was chosen as during the early years of adolescence many youth desire to learn how to drive and obtain their license so they can become more independent, as this is expected in our culture. It can serve as a catalyst to evoke memories of events that were attended and relationships that were forged away from home when engaged in activities with friends and peers. A final example is a photograph of empty chairs in Chapter 17, Death. Here, the intent was to represent the loss of loved ones, to evoke memories of past relationships, and to assist clients to reminisce about those they have lost. So when clients are viewing these photographs, encourage them to engage in creative interpretation and to let their imaginations guide them on a journey of discovery of their inner-most, subjective thoughts.

Glossary, Finally, a glossary of important terms, concepts, and processes discussed in this book has been included. Here, current definitions and interpretations are provided. This serves as a convenient source of pertinent information for therapists, clients, families, professors, students, and other professionals for whom this text is relevant.

Therapeutic Storytelling for Adolescents and Young Adults

1

Instructional Guidelines and Strategies

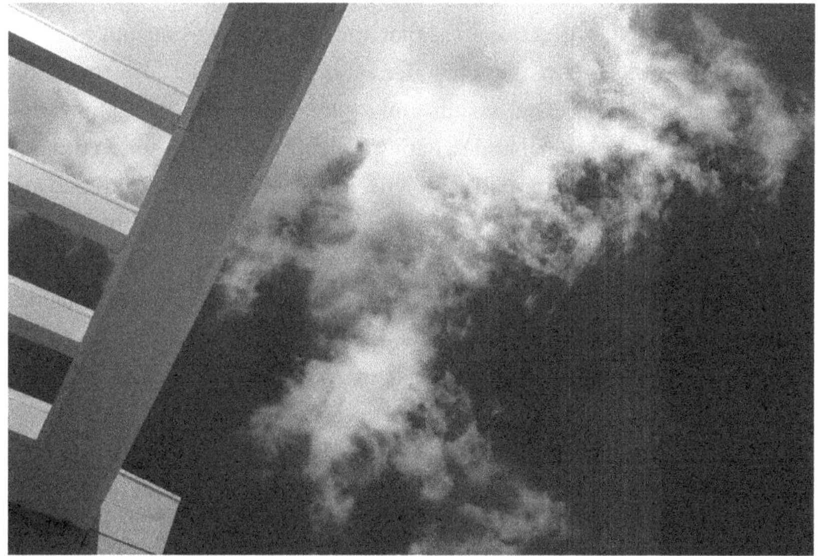

This book is designed to enhance the practical skills of mental health professionals through the creation and application of storytelling, narrative, writing, and other artistic endeavors. These forms of artistic expression assist and enable individuals to explore and further delve into life's challenges and triumphs. By further examination of self and others through use of verse and other visual and creative arts, one can promote healing and growth toward building a lifetime of resilience. The following passage from Mury Rabin's book *Art Therapy and Eating Disorders* eloquently describes the qualities and benefits of artistic expression of any type:

> *Art, whatever form it takes—a painting, a story, a poem, a musical composition, a dance—is always a product of the total being who creates it. It incorporates all of that artist's inner experiences as well as his multiple environments, including all the people who have been on the landscape of his life: his family and his world. All the good and nurturing things are there and all the negative and challenging experiences as well. They enter the prism of his life force and emerge alchemized in his unique vision. Each expands and humbles at the same time (Rabin, 2003, p. ix).*

Professionals reading this book will be able to build upon their own knowledge and theoretical perspectives regarding traditional talk therapy and expressive arts techniques. In addition to the knowledge gained, the easily accessible creative arts and storytelling activities and worksheets provided in this book and the accompanying website will enhance the challenging work of the busy mental health professional. Brief reviews of important materials benefit professionals as well as clients.

A practitioner using this book will be able to turn to a section as needed and find the desired area of practice that is best suited to a given client's needs, challenges, or strengths. The book is arranged by key practice areas that are relevant to the various needs of adolescents and young adults today. These practice areas include social adjustment and peer acceptance; sexuality; abuse, sexual assault, and exploitation; parental relationships; relationships; eating issues; emotional issues; dating violence; substance abuse; trauma; military issues; grief; strengths; community violence; independence; cultural and religious issues; job loss and poverty; illness and disability; school issues; and so forth.

Teens and young adults in therapy may identify with these reality-based stories to enable them to work through challenging situations in their lives. They may serve as springboards for discussion and development of positive, healthy goal setting and action plans for the future. Individuals may also write their own endings to stories pertinent to their life challenges. Increased emotional self-expression may occur as teens and young adults discuss, write, draw, paint, utilize drama, sing, or compose music as expressive means of formulating endings to stories and situations pertinent to their own lives.

Gradual Self-Disclosure Storytelling Technique

The stories provided in this book serve as a therapeutic base for interactive discussions between the practitioner and client. One way to utilize the stories in therapy is to have the clients finish the endings to stories by talking about, writing about, or drawing their own endings. The Gradual Self-Disclosure Storytelling Technique uses four distinct levels of inquiry to assist clients who are uncomfortable with self-disclosure.

Level-one questions enable clients to simply answer questions regarding characters in the story. It is hoped that clients will identify with characters' situations and gain insight into themselves through this experience. Level-two questions are written in such a manner that individuals may answer questions relating to someone other than themselves, such as a friend or family member, who has had experiences similar to characters in the story. This allows for slightly more disclosure from the client. Level-three questions directly address emotional issues relevant to the client's life by asking specifically about how the client's situation is similar to the situation of the story's characters. This level requires even more disclosure from the teen or young adult regarding his or her own life. Level-four requires the highest level of disclosure. The individual is asked to finish the ending to his or her own story by writing about, talking about, or drawing the ending.

Customization of Stories

Stories may be customized to meet the individualized needs of clients. By using the accompanying website, practitioners may personalize activity sheets by changing details of stories, adding clients' names, or altering situations. These personalized stories and activities may then be printed for direct use by the client. When working with adolescents and young adults, the stories may be customized in the following ways to meet the highly individualized needs of clients:

- Include the name of the teen or young adult on personalized stories and activities.
- Include the names of friends, family members, and pets when appropriate.
- Include the names of boyfriends or girlfriends.
- Change the gender of story characters.
- Alter the culture or cultural context of characters in the stories.
- Add details about the individual teen or young adult, such as eye color, hair color, if glasses are worn, type of clothing worn, personality traits, and so forth.
- Include activities or hobbies that teens or young adults may enjoy and participate in such as football, dance, track, speech team, band, philanthropic or character building clubs, youth or religious groups, and so forth.
- Add details about places and events that have been or are central to the adolescent's or young adult's life, such as schools or universities attended, places of worship, communities, birthdays, pertinent anniversaries, and so on.
- Incorporate particular strengths and challenges of characters into the plot of a story to more closely mirror an individual's life circumstances.
- Insert photographs of the individual, friends, or family members onto the story page when deemed appropriate.
- Insert clip art or Internet photographs that depict interests of the teen or young adult such as depictions of musicians, bands, actors, actresses, artists, and the like.

Visual Artistic Expression

Other modes of artistic expression may also be incorporated in a complementary fashion to enhance expression of emotions within the context of storytelling. A creative method of treatment, phototherapy, or using photos to draw out cognitions, emotions, and client narratives serves as a complementary expressive arts media. Photos in and associated with this book and website serve as springboards for therapeutic conversations, and depict a point of departure to delve deeper into clients' thoughts, feelings, and narratives.

Art may convey and reveal subtle shades of meaning and elucidate client-centered narratives and stories. Through painting, with brushes or with the fingers, one may allow for more complete release of authentic emotions through representation of feelings through interpretation of colors. Mardie Rossi and Karen Mackie describe this when discussing their exercise, the "Feelings Landscape" in which individuals, including adolescents and adults are encouraged to finger paint in order to explore various emotional states of being. They encourage their clients to "put their feelings into words by speaking from the colors (e.g., I am yellow and I feel ashamed. I am very big and am always here.)" (2011, p. 97).

In an existential sense, this type of artistic expression can contribute to making meaning of one's own existence. In this sense, therapists may engage individuals to ponder their place within the scope of their broader world and consider the impact their decisions have upon their world (Mannion, 2011). This may be particularly relevant to working with those in adolescence and young adulthood, as they tend to seek out why they are who they are and attempt to discover all of the possibilities of the person that they may become. Their artwork may function as a reflection, concrete representation, or illumination of their personal narratives.

Art facilitates communication more readily than words for some individuals who have difficulty expressing themselves verbally. Accessing and processing of painful emotions may occur through the creation of personalized artwork or creative activity. Many clients may feel safer and less afraid to express themselves when using drawing, painting, or sculpting than when engaged in more traditional types of talk therapies. Through art, individuals may gain understanding and insight into themselves and others (Malchiodi, 2003).

Of course, art is essential in the work of art therapists. However, many other types of therapists may benefit from incorporating aspects of art therapy into their practice. Others who may utilize artistic expression in assessment and treatment of clients include "clinical counselors, social workers, play therapists, marriage and family therapists, psychologists, and psychiatrists" (Malchiodi, 2003, p. xiii).

When referring to therapeutic artwork, Roberta Nadeau recommends that therapists facilitate "the reawakening of inner self" and "begin to encourage expressions of truth and personal satisfaction" (2008, p. 52). She also acknowledges that individuals may need to be gently prodded or encouraged to participate, especially if they are unaccustomed to the freedom allowed through artistic expression. If people feel they are not artistic, instead of presenting them with numerous modalities or mediums of expression such as pastels, oil paints, charcoal, and so forth, it may be better and more appropriate to begin in a simple manner. For those afraid of artistic expression, it may be suitable to suggest that they simply draw with a pencil onto a plain sheet of paper (Nadeau, 2008).

Art therapy has been shown to be an effective means of treatment for teenagers experiencing depression (Connor, 2002). One reason is that many adolescents will act out when depressed. Examples of acting-out behaviors may include drug or alcohol use, hitting walls, driving recklessly, or indiscriminant sexual behavior. Excessive anger may also be present, which may contribute to delinquent behaviors and parental conflicts. It is theorized that utilizing art as a means of therapy may benefit depressed adolescents who act out partially because it is a therapy involving activity instead of passivity (Riley, 2003).

The artwork itself may be used in an interesting therapeutic manner. Adolescents may often avoid direct eye contact with the therapist, however: "By averting the gaze from eye to eye to eye to art, a midplace has been created" (Riley, 2003, p. 226), which is safe for both. The artwork may serve as a buffer between the therapist and client, as both may look directly at the art, instead of at each other. Discussion may focus on the artwork, relieving pressure for the adolescent by not expecting him or her to directly talk about uncomfortable personal issues. This increases feelings of control and power in the teen (Riley, 2003). In a sense, clients' stories may be told and heard in a nonverbal fashion through their creation of narrative-related art. Lifemaps, in which clients draw or write the stories of their lives, may be beneficial.

In general, Riley has identified four positive aspects of art therapy that benefit adolescent clients. First, the clients exercise some control over how they communicate in therapy. This ability to choose what they draw and what they discuss potentially empowers them. Second, teens may benefit because they perceive feelings of respect from the therapist, especially if the practitioner finds value in the artwork of the clients. Third, teens have the chance to experience a sense of omnipotence through creativity and artistic expression. They have the opportunity to direct and be in charge of their own projects. Idealism may be expressed, as well as criticisms of parents, teachers, and friends, without fear of repercussions. Fourth, externalization of problematic situations or circumstances may occur through creation of real artwork that reflects inner psychic challenges or outer situational and environmental difficulties. The material or physical product allows for distancing from problems and reevaluation of situations. Individuals may also alter artistic work as a potentially safe precursor to changing their lives in the real world (Riley, 2003). This type of externalization of problems is similar to performing verbal components of narrative therapy techniques.

When integrating art creatively with psychotherapy it "must be recognized as a vital component of life, across time and cultures. Art has the same goals as therapy: communication, catharsis, appreciation of life in all its dimensions, the expression of values and beliefs, and in non-Western forms of therapy, affirmation of spirituality" (Coleman & Farris-Dufrene, 1996, p. 15). Additional methods of using therapeutic narrative and storytelling are further explored in the chapters that follow.

Additional Resources

Malchiodi, C. A. (2007). *The art therapy sourcebook.* New York: McGraw-Hill.

Morgan, A. (2000). *What is narrative therapy? An easy-to-read introduction.* Adelaide, South Australia: Dulwich Centre.

Slivinske, J., & Slivinske, L. (2011). *Storytelling and other activities for children in therapy.* Hoboken, NJ: John Wiley & Sons.

White, M. (2007). *Maps of narrative practice.* New York: W. W. Norton.

2

Conceptual Framework and Evidence-Based Practice

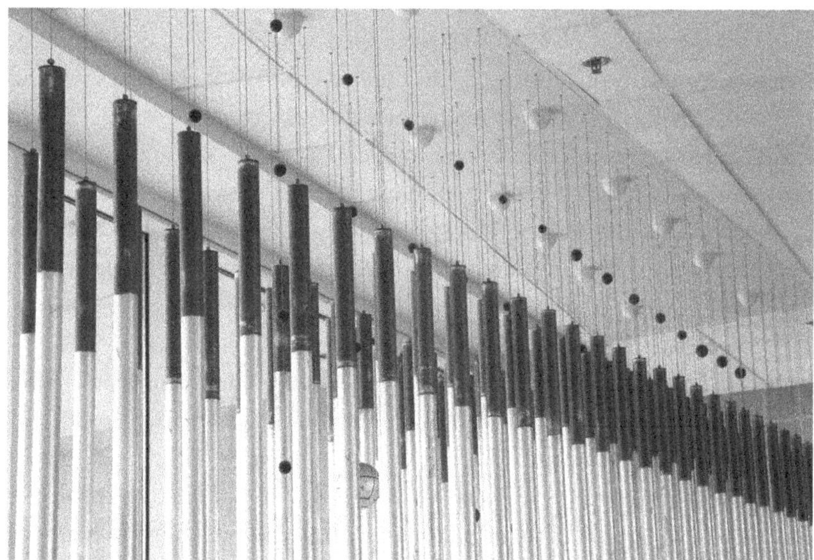

The conceptual framework used in this book is based upon a number of major tenets of Richard Gardner's mutual storytelling technique (1970, 1971, 1972, 1974), Michael White and David Epston's narrative therapy (1990, 2004, 2007), and the strengths-based perspective of Dennis Saleebey (2002). Gardner (1974) believes that storytelling can be practiced therapeutically to treat children with a variety of psychogenic problems. He describes his technique as a method of communication at the patient's own level. The therapist, with the client, upon hearing the story selects important themes, uses the same characters, and creates a story that has more positive adaptations and outcomes. Gardner believes this approach avoids the anxiety produced by other, more directive, types of therapy and can be used to elucidate the norms, values, and beliefs of society so that patients may gain more insight into the issues they face. White and Epston (1990) developed a form of psychotherapy that employs narrative as a major component of their method. They conceptualize that the story told by the person in therapy is an important mechanism through which a person can express a variety of problems. This method applies therapeutic questioning to enable clients to identify important issues and then assist them in reformulating more positive directions and outcomes to their situations (Shapiro & Ross, 2002). After the story is told the therapist facilitates deconstructing their story by assigning meaning and guiding them in the externalization or objectification of the problem. In this fashion, the therapist helps individuals see that they are not the problem but that the problem in and of itself is the problem. So the problem becomes a major focus of treatment. Also, the therapist assists the clients in retelling their stories by helping them identify intentions, hopes, dreams, and strengths to develop a more positive direction in life. In this way, the therapist encourages people to use their beliefs, knowledge, and skills in regaining their lives from their problems. The problem is placed outside the person and inside the culture. In other words, the contexts in which problems are located are examined and the role of society in creating or maintaining the problems is explored (Etchison & Kleist, 2000). Finally, Dennis Saleebey posits that clients may access their strengths through the application of storytelling. Types of strengths related stories include personal and family tales, folklore, and cultural stories. As clients and therapists together make meaning of these stories and experiences, clients can access valuable lessons learned, strengths, and gain insight. Various types of stories promote change and healing, including those of resistance, challenge, struggle, resilience, and oppression. Saleebey also promotes highlighting a client's gifts, assets, and strengths in general (Saleebey, 1997).

Our framework builds on and extends these ideas. Our concept is similar to Gardner's in that stories are told and retold, at times with the help of a therapist. Retelling stories with clients empowers and challenges them to look toward possibilities in altering their thinking and perception, as well as the possibility of making positive change. Themes of safety and comfort may be built into stories, and more positive outcomes and adaptations can be integrated throughout. Our concept differs in that it is more directive; the role of the therapist is vital in directing the initial story selection based on the mental health needs of the particular client. In addition, our Gradual Self-Disclosure Storytelling Technique allows clients to express their stories through a variety of media. Their stories may be told through verbal means, through drawing or types of artwork, or through writing.

Our conceptual framework is similar to White and Epston's work insofar as it addresses externalization of the problem, albeit in a unique manner. By reading or being told a specific story about a person with a problem similar to their own, clients may distance themselves enough from the problem insomuch as this actually enables them to gain access to it. Through the externalization or distancing, a clearer, less subjective perspective may be acquired. We include questions after each topical story that reflect four levels of disclosure, with level-one requiring the least amount of disclosure and level-four the most. The problem is also externalized though the accompanying story questions at levels-one and two and in the corresponding worksheets. Employing our Gradual Self-Disclosure Storytelling Technique involves four graduated levels of questioning and client self-disclosure. At level-one, clients are asked direct questions about characters in the story and their problems, thus allowing for externalization and distancing from their own problems. At level-two, clients are asked questions regarding "someone they know" who may have a similar problem, allowing for some proximity to the problem while still maintaining externalization and distancing. We also promote deconstruction and reconstruction of the story, with positive, adaptive outcomes integrated throughout the reconstructed narrative. Our concept differs in that clients are directed toward specific stories based on identified needs and therapist assessment. It also differs insomuch as four distinct levels of disclosure are available to assist clients in the restorying process. Also, our technique allows for multiple media of story expression, including verbal narrative, art, and written expression.

Finally, our framework integrates concepts of Saleebey's strengths perspective in both the text and story questions. It examines how to elicit strengths from and with clients through careful and thoughtful questioning and strengths assessment. In addition, strengths are elicited from clients in the restorying process by promoting the positive aspects of one's life, including strengths of community, self, family, and peers. It encourages clients to tell their stories, as does the strengths perspective. Our approach provides a more concrete and accessible format for them to readily tell their stories through a variety of means, including the oral tradition, through art, or through the written word.

Efficacy Evidence to Guide Practice

The effectiveness of narrative therapy practices has been examined in a number of qualitative and quantitative research studies. Seymour and Epston (1989), in their study of 45 cases of childhood stealing, used therapeutic mapping in their therapy sessions. They found that six to twelve months after therapy, 80% of the children no longer stole or had substantially reduced rates of stealing. Besa (1994) studied the effectiveness of components of narrative therapy in reducing parent-child conflicts in six families with children ranging in age from 8 to 17 years. Multiple baseline designs were employed that investigated the target behaviors of arguing, not doing homework, not doing chores, and the like which were producing the conflicts. Analysis of their data revealed that five of the six families had an 88% to 98% reduction in parent-childhood conflicts as a result of narrative therapy. They noted that these decreased rates only occurred in the presence of narrative therapy and were not observed in its absence. In a study by St-James-O'Connor, Meakes, Pickering, and Schuman (1997), an ethnographic research design was used to analyze the perceptions and meanings eight families with children had regarding their experience with narrative therapy. The presenting problems included family violence, divorce, death, attention deficit/hyperactivity disorder, failure to obey rules and direction, and other conduct disorders. Through a standardized interview format the researchers questioned families and identified major themes from their data. They concluded that these themes were consistent with the view that narrative therapy empowered family members in their striving to change. It was further observed that all families reported a reduction in family problems and that the reduction was greater for families that were involved with narrative therapy for longer periods than those involved for shorter periods.

In 1998, Silver, Williams, Worthington, and Phillips conducted a retrospective study of narrative therapy outcomes for 108 children with soiling problems. Fifty-four children were treated using narrative therapy's externalization, while the comparison group of 54 were treated using the traditional methods of therapy employed at the same clinic. The outcomes for the narrative therapy group were better than those exposed to traditional therapy. Also, the parents at follow-up rated externalization as being more helpful than the other methods. In an exploratory, descriptive study by Weston, Boxer, and Heatherington (1998), 92 children and their families were appraised. These researchers, with the intent of increasing understanding of the children's cognitions, studied the attributions children attached to stories about the causes of family arguments. Children were randomly assigned to two treatment conditions. One group heard an audiotaped argument between a parent and a parent, while the other group heard one between a parent and a child. These tapes served as a stimulus to recall real arguments that occurred in their family setting. Five structured interview instruments and a pictorial scale were used to gather data, which included the children's perceptions of arguments between parents, arguments between parents and children, and their affect. Data were analyzed using a repeated-measures ANOVA. The authors concluded that use of creative informational strategies such as storytelling and props were more useful than other methods. They also believed that appreciating children's stories and the associated attributions of the causes of family conflict can benefit the entire family when using narrative therapy.

In an exploratory study of eight families treated by eight therapists, Coulehan, Friedlander, and Heatherington (1998) attempted to reveal the components of the change process involved in the families' successful transformation of narratives. Children in this study had multiple problems, such as violence, eating disorders, failure in the school setting, noncompliance with rules, removal from the home, and so forth. All therapists were trained regarding the use of narrative therapy. Successful outcomes were thought to occur when transformations such as new experiences, actions, and meanings were associated with the original family stories. Families' postsession questionnaires were administered to parents and to the therapists. The qualitative method of constant comparison was used to analyze the data collected. Successful and unsuccessful therapy sessions were compared. These researchers concluded that they had support for the efficacy in the use of the narrative approach.

Muntigl (2004) explored how the narrative therapy process enables client change. In this case study, six sessions using narrative therapy were extensively examined. It was determined that at the end of therapy the client was able to produce narratives that displayed positive change and self-control. A paper by Weber, Davis, and McPhie (2006) analyzed seven depressed women who participated in a weekly group for 10 weeks that used narrative therapy. Pretest, posttest comparisons revealed that there was a reduction in depression scores and the risk of eating disorders. They concluded that narrative therapy resulted in these positive changes. In 2011, Vromans and Schweitzer investigated the use of narrative therapy with 47 adults who were experiencing depression. After eight sessions of narrative therapy, posttherapy outcomes showed an improvement in depressive symptoms. The proportion of clients that showed reliable improvement was 74%, while those achieving clinically significant improvement was 53%. A 3-month follow-up revealed that the depressive symptom reduction was maintained.

Qualitatively, we have witnessed the transformation of adolescents and young adults who have benefitted from our therapeutic process. Our methods have enabled them to further self-disclose, especially those who are socially awkward or inhibited. It also has promoted discussion surrounding sensitive issues such as sexual assault and abuse and has furthered the development of rapport. Others have identified with oppositional behaviors of story characters, which has allowed for conversations surrounding consequences for destructive behaviors and more socially acceptable alternatives. Many have benefitted by being encouraged to tell their own stories, as evidenced by decreases in destructive habits; improved relationships with peers, teachers, siblings, and parents; and fewer expulsions from the school setting.

We conducted a focus group of young adults in a class at their university. The young adults were asked to discuss various aspects of storytelling and the therapeutic relationship. Of the 23 individuals in the focus group, 19 participants responded that they do identify with and relate to characters in stories. One young male adult stated that when he first joined Alcoholics' Anonymous, he was directed to read stories about people who had experienced alcoholism and who had experienced challenges and successes in their recovery. He believed that this power of storytelling helped him to self-disclose, "broke down his walls," and motivated him to change. He now incorporates stories into the help he gives to others in recovery, as he is now a sponsor for other young men. This particular man felt that "realistic stories" could help people to break their "codes of silence" regarding their problems. A young woman stated that she felt that the expressive arts, including writing about herself, was an enjoyable activity that she participated in while a high school student. This experience helped her gain increased insight about herself while an adolescent. Another young woman supported the idea of using storytelling and other types of activities in therapy with teenagers, as she has four of her own children who are currently in therapy. She feels that storytelling and other types of therapeutic activities would be useful to help them to "open up" and feel relaxed with their therapists. Nine young adults felt that they would benefit from storytelling and other types of activities to help to "draw them out" or assist them in the process of therapeutic self-disclosure, instead of just directly talking to the therapist. Those who were more socially inhibited appeared more likely to benefit from interventions involving storytelling and other types of activities while in the therapeutic relationship. Another young woman felt that stories could benefit teens and young adults by teaching them appropriate societal expectations, such as how to prepare for and how to behave in a job interview. She expressed her opinion that some people are not taught or prepared for this type of professional interaction. She felt that through storytelling, appropriate social skills could be learned and applied.

A convenience sample of two classes was also selected and administered an appreciation of storytelling questionnaire by the authors. Of the 53 participants, 40 were young adults with an average age of 24.3. Of these 40, 15% were male and 85% were female; 42.5% resided in the city, 45% lived in suburbs, and the remaining 12.5% lived in rural areas; 42.6% were in the lower income bracket and 53.8% indicated they had middle incomes. Regarding race, 72.5% were white, while 27.5% were African American. The questionnaire contained a 13 item Likert type scale that measured their appreciation of storytelling in a therapeutic setting. The theoretical range of the scale was 13–65, with high scores indicating the greatest appreciation. The internal consistency of the scale was examined and considered to be acceptable as Cronbach's alpha was found to be .73. The content and discriminant validity of the scale also were investigated and thought to be satisfactory. Eighty percent of the respondents agreed or strongly agreed that all important aspects of storytelling were included, while the discriminant check revealed that significantly different mean scale scores were obtained when the upper and lower quartile scale scores of the scale were compared using an independent samples t-test ($mean_{Q1} = 44.8$ and $mean_{Q4} = 58.2$, $t = -11.667$, d.f. $= 9.717$, $p = .000$). The average scale score for participants was 53, indicating a high level of appreciation of storytelling as a therapeutic technique. Example items revealed that 85% agreed or strongly agreed they would feel comfortable reading a story and answering story questions about someone they did not know or who had a problem similar to theirs. Likewise 87.5% agreed or strongly agreed that once their real problem had been addressed they would feel comfortable rewriting or retelling the story with the aid of the therapist so that it had a more positive outcome. Finally, 92.5% agreed or strongly agreed that they believed that storytelling is a useful therapeutic technique for adolescents and young adults.

Additional Resources

Etchison, M., & Kleist, D. M. (2000). Review of narrative therapy: Research and utility. *The Family Journal: Counseling and Therapy for Couples and Families*, 8(1), 61–66.

Gardner, R. A. (1971). *Therapeutic communication with children: The mutual storytelling technique.* New York: Science House.

Saleebey, D. (2002). *The strengths perspective in social work practice* (3rd ed.). Boston, MA: Allyn & Bacon.

White, M. (2004). *Narrative practice and exotic lives: Resurrecting diversity in everyday life.* Adelaide, South Australia: Dulwich Centre Publications.

White, M. (2007). *Maps of narrative practice.* New York: W. W. Norton

White, M., & Epston, D. (1990). *Narrative means to therapeutic ends.* New York: W. W. Norton.

3

Principles and Processes of Storytelling with Teens and Young Adults

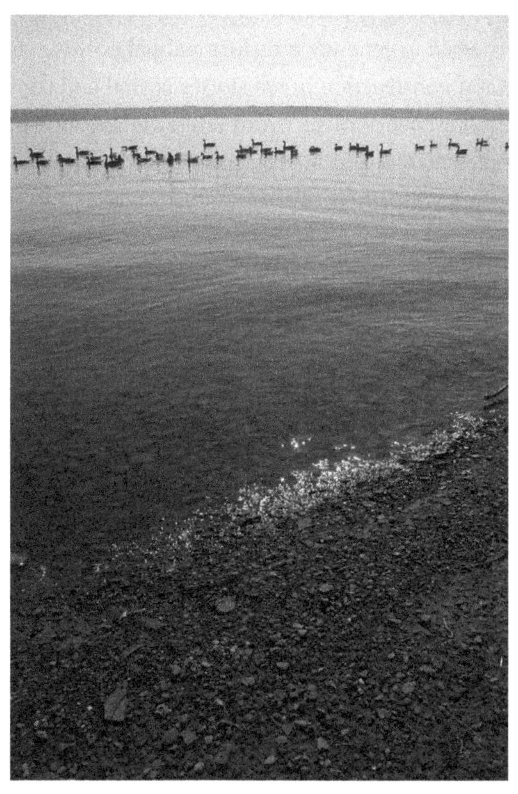

One method of reaching and helping people in need is through the telling of stories. Stories represent and reflect cultural beliefs and values, as well as morals affecting decision making and rules and laws. Stories have been told throughout history to influence and change human behavior through insight gained and lessons learned (Erford, Eaves, Bryant, & Young, 2010).

Storytelling has been found to be an effective method of reaching adolescents and young adults, especially with those individuals for whom direct expression of emotions is difficult. Through storytelling, one may relate to and identify with characters in stories, which at times may seem less threatening than directly discussing personal matters about one's life. When a person feels ready, he or she may then begin to divulge more about himself or herself. Lessons learned about fictitious characters may then be applied to real-life circumstances and situations.

Storytelling comes naturally to many people, and it often is relied on as a learning tool within educational systems. It is also an important medium for transmitting information, values, and morals from one generation to the next within the context of immediate and extended familial relationships. Historically speaking, cultural and ethnic traditions and strengths have been passed down in this manner, often involving the oral tradition of storytelling. Stories may be so powerful that they evoke strong emotions in the listener, reader, or author of the stories. It is suggested that when this occurs, these strong emotions and insights gained be harnessed to generate transformational positive change in people's lives.

In narrative therapy, construction of life stories is vital and contributes to our understanding of the self and our environment. Word usage and creation of life stories formulate and contribute to people's mental and interpersonal worlds. Personal stories influence our lives, as do our interactions with others, and these stories and narratives impact understanding of self. Life narratives affect human beings' perceptions of self, in both detrimental and helpful ways, dependent on internal story lines. One technique useful in storytelling and the narrative process is that "Through a process of refocusing, practitioners help clients to construct different life narratives that portray them in a different light" (Walsh, 2007, p. 111).

In adolescence individuals may begin to be able to step back from themselves and write autobiographically, when and if ready. An alternative perspective for them to take when doing this is to write about their lives in the third person. It may allow them to gain a unique perspective about their own lives that they may have otherwise missed. They may be more willing to identify the strengths and weaknesses of themselves when viewed through the lens of an observer or formulator of characters within a story (Wanner, 1994). Level-four activities within this book would allow teens and young adults to express themselves in an autobiographical sense, if desired.

Writing and drawing may benefit adolescents in treatment by promoting self-disclosure and self-discovery (DeLucia-Waack, 2006). Stories and activities should be selected that are pertinent to the needs of those in treatment. This will enable individuals to relate to the situational issues and plots of characters. Clients may then be able to relate to and identify with characters, vicariously express emotions, and problem-solve based on characters' stories. Ideally, clients will eventually be empowered to share their own personal narratives.

In addition, adolescents and young adults may be able to successfully develop positive self-concepts through writing or telling stories about themselves. Crawford, Brown, and Crawford suggest that a "person's identity is created rather than revealed through narrative" (2004, p. 110). They also discuss another way of using stories to help individuals regarding identity formation: stories may be used by individuals to form "more effective, competent, and even pleasurable identities" (2004, p. 110).

Through the art of storytelling, adolescents and young adults may begin to feel less alone in their traumatic experiences and may gain insight into their own and others' behaviors, thoughts, and emotions. By expressing themselves through writing, verbal storytelling, and artistic means such as painting, drawing, and sculpting, teens and young adults may release painful or confusing emotions in a supportive therapeutic environment. Other expressive arts modalities may also be used, such as drama therapy, phototherapy, songwriting, and other musical or dance interventions. These means of self-expression may serve as a springboard for planning, goal setting, and positive change in the lives of adolescents and young adults. This is crucial during these developmental stages, which lay the foundation for so much of a positive, well-adjusted adulthood.

Adolescents may be more likely to engage and invest in therapy through the use of expressive or creative arts than through more traditional modes of treatment, such as having typical conversations with a therapist. Another benefit of using the creative arts with adolescents is that teens may produce something tangible that they can keep, share, and reflect upon (DeLucia-Waack, 2006). When using the activities and stories in this book, adolescents may choose to keep or share their stories, drawings, or paintings.

It is imperative when practicing therapeutic storytelling to instruct individuals to allow themselves to be creative. Let them know that they will not be judged for the quality of their writing, drawing, painting, and so forth. Tell them that it is not important if words are misspelled or if drawings are artistically constructed. What is important is that they express themselves in an open and free manner so as to allow the therapist to assist them with the personal issues that may be troubling them. Of course, expression of happiness and joy are equally important for resilience and growth of adolescent and young adult clients.

Role-plays may benefit adolescents and young adults in treatment, and stories may be acted out with assistance from a therapist in a group setting where characters are assigned or with family members. In the context of groups for adolescents, those conducting the groups may "provide scenarios and roles for group members, and include coaching to increase risk taking and trying out of new behaviors" (DeLucia-Waack, 2006, p. 155). Experimentation with new or familiar situations, emotions, and behaviors may occur in this milieu in a relatively safe environment. Through role-playing stories, valuable insights may be gained that may lead to behavioral change that may then be applied to individuals' own lives and circumstances.

The effectiveness of therapeutic writing has been demonstrated in various situations. Expressive writing can be successfully applied among a variety of population groups. It may be used with clients who may be experiencing typical developmental crises or issues. Those who have experienced traumatic events in their lives may benefit as well. It has been implemented successfully with those who suffer from serious illnesses and those who were traumatized by terrorist attacks. Writings of these types may involve the mental health practitioner prompting or starting the writing session (Degges-White, 2011). In this book, therapeutic stories and story-starters are provided to aid the client and practitioner in initiating the writing process. Stories may then be completed or rewritten either in session or as homework assignments when appropriate.

Components of narrative therapy may also benefit a variety of people with disabilities and mental or physical challenges. In fact, according to Cashin, adolescents living with various forms of autism, including Asperger's Disorder, may benefit from narrative approaches to treatment. He refers to this paradoxical appearance by stating that "Although epistemologically incongruent with what would be expected to be of use in work with someone with autism, the tools used in narrative therapy provide the platform for a novelly successful and changing approach to psychotherapy with such less typical thinkers" (Cashin, 2008, p. 52). Concrete visual artwork and story writing techniques utilized throughout this text may benefit those with autism by allowing them to visually experience their stories in a tangible, concrete manner. In addition, unproductive, cyclical narratives may be deconstructed and reconstructed to promote positive outcomes for teens with autism (Cashin, 2008).

Another effective method when using storytelling involves use of the "Progressive Story" (Divinyi, 1995). With this technique, individuals build upon a story, further developing the plot and adding characters if desired. They may learn vicariously from the experiences of characters in the story. For example, if characters make positive decisions, the teens and adults building the story may be more likely to choose positive life decisions as well. If negative choices are made by the characters, the story builders may see the repercussions, such as possible drug addiction, jail time, or relationship consequences, and learn lessons that can be applied to their own lives (Divinyi, 1995).

Healing stories may also be used therapeutically with individuals. Stories may be written and rewritten, with or without the practitioner's help, as a means of reframing potential challenges or life stories in clients' lives. Through this process of reframing, fresh and insightful perspectives may be gained, and teens and young adults may begin to feel empowered in this process of growth. Through reframing and rewriting stories, individuals have the opportunity for recreating meaning of previous or current life experiences. At times, strengths may be identified through this highly personalized experience (Slattery, 2004).

In addition, behaviors and ideations that are perhaps maladaptive or counterproductive may be recognized and reframed in treatment as ways of coping under difficult circumstances. This may contribute to feelings of empowerment through the potential realization of an internalized locus of control (Slattery, 2004). Breaking down, or deconstructing, fictitious or autobiographical stories and then rewriting or reconstructing them may be a powerful experience contributing to growth, healing, and feelings of control over one's environment and life.

When and if ready, individuals may decide to specifically tell the details of their own stories. When divulging their life stories, bear in mind that stories will vary depending on various factors occurring at that given point in time. Their stories in a sense represent a "snapshot" in time based on their perception of events, differences in developmental levels, and views of self. Of course, the cultural and situational content and context of individuals' stories should be considered within the therapeutic discourse and through the processing of information (Thomas & Schwarzbaum, 2011). At times, it may benefit the client if the therapist assists in the telling, or co-narration, of the story (Ferro, 2006).

Some practitioners may choose to focus on patterns or themes that emerge when clients tell or write their own narratives. Reflection of themes back to clients can be an important component of co-constructing their stories. These reflections can prove interesting to clients and provide the opportunity to gain insight into themselves and their life situations. The therapists' perspectives should be viewed as only one factor within the context of the therapeutic discourse, bearing in mind that therapists are influenced by their own worldviews and experiences (Lewis, 2007).

Another valuable technique, with permission, is that of restorying. In this process, the practitioner borrows another's story, and tells it when it is applicable to another person's life. Through restorying, one may gain insight into self and others and witness how positive resolutions regarding difficult situations were achieved (Lewis, 2007). In certain circumstances, it may also be appropriate to borrow stories from the practitioners' own lives, when it would benefit the adolescents and young adults with whom they are working. For example, a professional could share a story about how she resolved a disagreement she had with her own parents regarding school conflicts, privileges, or dating issues.

Families, as well as individuals, also have their own unique stories to tell. Events within the family system are experienced differently by each member. By telling their stories, families may view situations from different perspectives, and problems may become externalized. The family member may not be viewed as the problem, but the behaviors of the member may be problematic. Negative family narratives may be rewritten in a positive manner to benefit family members and encourage growth and development (Nichols & Schwartz, 2006).

Additional Resources

Crenshaw, D. A. (2008). *Therapeutic engagement of children and adolescents: Play, symbol, drawing, and storytelling strategies.* Plymouth, UK: Aronson.

Gardner, R. A. (1971). *Therapeutic communication with children: The mutual storytelling technique.* New York: Science House.

Slivinske, J., & Slivinske, L. (2011). *Storytelling and other activities for children in therapy.* Hoboken, NJ: John Wiley & Sons.

White, M. (2000). *Reflections on narrative practice.* Adelaide, South Australia: Dulwich Centre Publications.

White, M. (2004). *Narrative practice and exotic lives: Resurrecting diversity in everyday life.* Adelaide, South Australia: Dulwich Centre Publications.

White, M., & Morgan, A. (2006). *Narrative therapy with children and their families.* Adelaide, South Australia: Dulwich Centre Publications.

White, M. (2007). *Maps of narrative practice.* New York: W. W. Norton.

4

Developmental Issues of Adolescence and Young Adulthood

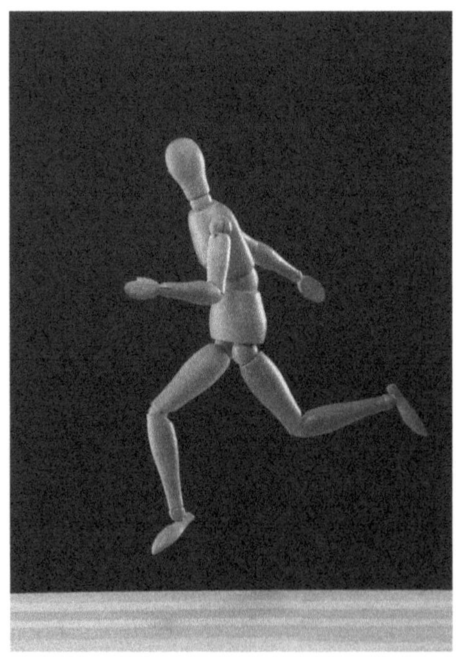

Adolescence and young adulthood may be a confusing and tumultuous time for many individuals. For others, it may be a joyous, carefree period of life. This book was written with the needs, challenges, hopes, and strengths of these age groups in mind. When utilizing the information, stories, and activities throughout this book, it is imperative to remain cognizant of the developmental levels and issues of various clients.

During adolescence, teens will encounter several physiological changes. These include the development of secondary sex characteristics such as the growth of facial and pubic hair, breast development, deepening of the voice, and so forth. Females may begin their menstrual cycles, if this has not already occurred in middle childhood. Also, hormonal fluctuations may contribute to increases in moodiness, feelings of sadness or sullenness, as well as aggressive or acting-out behaviors.

Teens may experience concerns regarding changes occurring in their bodies. They may become mildly or greatly upset over the development of acne, about gaining weight or obesity, and about whether they are developing early or late. Boys who develop early generally tend to feel better about themselves, and they tend to be more athletic, have better friendships, and tend to feel increased confidence. However, girls who develop earlier tend to encounter more challenges academically and behaviorally, and may feel poorly about their physical appearance (Ashford & LeCroy, 2010). Bear in mind that these generalizations will not apply to everyone, and each individual's circumstances, levels of social support, strengths, and type of personality merit consideration and mediate how early maturation may affect any one person.

Adolescents and young adults may struggle with attempts to formulate their own identity. This is a typical and expected part of development, especially within the context of Western cultural expectations. Adolescents may distance themselves from parents or caregivers in order to further the development of self. This "breaking away" or individuation may contribute to adolescent and parental conflicts, particularly when teens and parents hold incongruent beliefs and value systems. Adolescents and young adults may experiment with various life roles, which, one hopes, will contribute to a permanent "finding" of the self—discovering who one is. This commonly is referred to as identity formation.

In Western culture, adolescence and young adulthood are periods in which separation from parents is often encouraged. Young people may move away from home or attend college in another city or state, distant from immediate family members. Experiencing additional developmental challenges or struggles such as grief and mourning during this critical period may further encumber this difficult process of transition (Blundell, 2001). Those who do not establish some form of adequate independence may be viewed punitively.

Most conflicts between parents and adolescents involve disagreements or points of contention surrounding common everyday occurrences. For example, it would be typical for family members to argue about commonplace issues such as performing chores or completing homework. For most families, conflict surrounding drug and alcohol abuse and sexuality are far less common (Levine & Munsch, 2011). However, these more serious conflicts do occur in many households, and such situations merit extra care and attention to promote positive and healthy resolution.

Having a strong and caring bond with parents during adolescence tends to serve as a protective factor. It is vital to not underestimate the importance of caring relationships in the lives of adolescents. Although they may act as though they do not need anyone or do not desire support from parents or parental figures, this is often not the case. Simply "being there" for them as a reliable, dependable, and caring adult can make a difference in their lives and foster positive mental health and resilience (Hair, Moore, Garrett, Ling, & Cleveland, 2008). Many times, parents, caregivers, and helpers do not need to be perfect—they just need to be accessible, decent, caring human beings who are available when needed by the teens and young adults in their lives.

Other adults in teenagers' and young adults' lives may significantly impact their development, positively or negatively. These may include grandparents, friends of the family, fictive kin, aunts and uncles, religious leaders, favorite teachers or coaches, and so forth. It is hoped that positive relationships from extended family and other supports assist in guiding individuals toward optimal development. Mental health practitioners may also protect and buffer at-risk young people during periods of vulnerability.

Although the process of self-discovery and exploration are typical in adolescent and young adult development, this sometimes contributes to high-risk behaviors involving sexuality, drug and alcohol use, and violence. Teens and young adults often are influenced by their peer groups and try to "fit in" with one particular group. An important part of development involves formation of a positive peer group identity. Ideally, friends and classmates will influence peers to participate in healthy activities such as athletics, academics, clubs, and civic organizations. These friends and activities may serve as buffers against the challenging realities of everyday life. They also may provide enjoyment, the opportunity for recreational activities, and the necessary social connections to meet and develop an intimate relationship.

Adolescents and young adults depend on one another for socialization and support in regard to dating relationships, friendships, and for academic guidance and support. Numerous salient life decisions that impact future lifestyle, career, and relationship issues are determined during these foundational stages of life. Many individuals will change academic majors and career paths several times as they experiment with who they are and who they desire to become in the future. Dating and friendship relations may be altered and rearranged in attempts to identify and solidify personal and professional systems of values and beliefs. Adolescents and young adults who are confronted with exceptional or multiple life stressors during these stages may encounter increased difficulty mastering typical developmental tasks, in addition to life's typical developmental crises.

However, the desire to be wanted and accepted by the group leaves teens and young adults vulnerable to negative peer group activities such as substance abuse, gangs and community violence, irresponsible sexuality, criminal behavior, and so forth. Individuals may be easily swayed toward negative behaviors in order to fulfill their need to "fit in." For many people, this can be a very difficult and challenging time of life, when extra support may be needed.

Sexuality is an important part of adolescence. As teenagers, many will experiment with various aspects of friendship, love, and sexuality. Although physically mature, teens may be unprepared emotionally and cognitively to handle the intense emotions that may accompany their relationships and sexual experiences (Carrell, 2000). They may experience confusion or embarrassment regarding sexuality, reproduction, birth control, or sexual orientation, and sometimes they may turn to caring adults or professionals for support, comfort, and advice.

Many teens and young adults may also be parents themselves. These young parents may benefit from advice, as well as concrete referrals and services, regarding how to balance home life, child care, high school, university studies or vocational training, and work. In addition, advice about parenting may be helpful for young, inexperienced parents, as well as referrals to reputable child care agencies and so forth.

Well-known theorist Erik Erikson describes in his psychosocial theory eight psychosocial stages and crises that individuals pass through in their lives. When referring to psychosocial crises, he viewed these as typical developmental challenges or conflicts that everyone maneuvers over the life course. After successfully meeting the demands of each given psychosocial crisis during childhood, an individual then encounters the psychosocial crisis of adolescence, or identity versus role confusion (Newman & Newman, 2012).

When faced with the psychosocial crisis of identity versus role confusion, an individual is confronted with establishing a firm identity, or finding out who one truly is. This entails discovering unknown or unexplored aspects of oneself. This may occur in the context of exploring and further identifying beliefs and values, especially in regard to religious beliefs, sexuality, career goals, and so forth. Adolescents often struggle with finding out who they are and how they fit into society (Sigelman & Rider, 2012).

Teens may experiment with various possible identities. Some may experience only minor struggles with identity formation, while others may experience great degrees of confusion, stress, and anxiety. Many variables affect how one passes through adolescence, including family structure and support, temperament, hormonal levels, and typical and nontypical developmental stressors. Each individual will have factors and influences unique to his or her own circumstances.

The next stage of development, young adulthood, involves the psychosocial crisis of intimacy versus isolation. During this stage, an individual struggles to solidify close relationships, including but not limited to those with intimate partners, friends, and family. The individual prepares for and possibly becomes firmly rooted in a committed relationship to meet the demands of the challenges of developing intimacy (Sigelman & Rider, 2012). According to Erikson, if a person successfully builds a close and trusting relationship with another person, then he or she has successfully overcome the psychosocial crisis of intimacy versus isolation. If a person is unable to achieve this, he or she may feel isolated and lonely, lacking close emotional contact in personal relationships (Newman & Newman, 2012).Issues of gender, culture, ethnicity, sexual orientation, and disability are inextricably woven into the brocade of human development, including during the life stages of adolescence and young adulthood. Our environments and experiences cannot be separated from the essence of the developing self. Also to deny the realities of oppression, prejudice, discrimination, as well as the numerous positive attributes of differences, is to deny the realities of one's existence.

Ideas regarding what it means to be male or female in a given family, organization, community, or society impact everyone's development, whether male or female. For example, gender, in many parts of the world, determines if, where, and when females may be educated. It may also affect others' rights, such as the right to vote, work, choose a mate, or drive a vehicle. Unfortunately, cultural mores about gender may limit women's access to vital resources in many parts of the world.

Culture and ethnicity also impact opportunities or impose limits on opportunities faced by those in adolescence and young adulthood. Examples of potential areas where people may face discrimination include encounters as youth attempt to gain employment or enter into meaningful careers. In addition, some still cope with prejudice when entering into dating relationships or marriage with someone of a different ethnicity.

Those who have alternative sexual orientations or beliefs may also encounter unique struggles and discriminatory practices in the context of development as a young man or woman. They may be ostracized by family or friends, encounter employment discrimination, and confront even harsher penalties, depending upon the societal context. Youth with membership in multiple groups who have been historically discriminated against are challenged with even more risk factors to overcome in their struggles to become well-adjusted young adults and members of their societies.

Physical and mental challenges involving illness and disability also affect how one is treated across the lifespan. If a young person is denied access to opportunities afforded to others or if appropriate accommodations are not provided, he or she may deal with increased difficulty, due to discrimination, in accomplishing the developmental tasks of educational growth and career achievement. Special concerns may also arise in regard to the establishment of intimacy as well.

All of these groups of individuals confront the risk of marginalization and oppression (Kirst-Ashman, 2011) that affects development and access to opportunity. These mezzo, macro, and exosystem factors merit consideration as influences affecting development of those with specific gender, cultural, ethnic, sexual orientation, and disability issues. Oppression, and the context of disempowerment and discrimination, cannot be erased or removed from the indelible, undeniable experiences of individuals' realities of existence during the growth phases of adolescence and young adulthood.

Technology and Development

Adolescents and young adults may at times feel unsure of themselves about where they fit in their families, with their peers, their schools, and within their communities. Modern influences of technological advancement are affecting their development and interactions within and among these groups. In many instances, they are depending much more on technology than in the past, which conceivably is contributing to less face-to-face communication and increased interaction via electronic media. These media include social networking sites, texting via cell phones, blogging, and so forth.

Communication via these means can be positive or negative, dependent upon the context of the situation. Difficulties may arise when those who suffer from social isolation in school or the community continue to have this experience magnified and amplified via social media. This may occur via cyber-bullying, online social neglect or invisibility, and loneliness felt when witnessing others' extremely active social lives on social media sites, thus further contributing to feelings of isolation compared to the lives of others. It may also bring forth or exacerbate preexisting predispositions toward depression or anxiety in those who are not well adapted in their peer oriented relationships.

Conversely, social media may enhance positive and healthy relationship development as well. Interactions that were once conducted by telephone conversations may now be done via virtual face-to-face communications, allowing for enhanced personal and intimate communication with family and friends living in distant places. Furthermore, positive peer support and encouraging posts on social media sites may serve to increase individuals' self-esteem and buffer them in a protective manner in times of distress (e.g. relationship break-ups, deaths of loved ones, academic stressors and pressures, and so forth). Positive peer pressure, whether virtual or in person, often influences people to continue their life trajectory toward a healthy, productive pathway in life.

Additional Resources

Hendry, L. B., & Kloep, M. (2012). *Adolescence and adulthood: Transitions and transformations.* Houndsmills, Basingstoke, UK: Palgrave Macmillan.

Hutchison, E. D. (2008). *Dimensions of human behavior: The changing life course* (3rd ed.). Thousand Oaks, CA: Sage.

Santrock, J. W. (2012). *Adolescence* (14th ed.). New York: McGraw-Hill.

Sigelman, C. K., & Rider, E. A. (2012). *Life-span human development* (7th ed.). Belmont, CA: Wadsworth.

5

The Strengths Approach to Storytelling with Adolescents and Young Adults

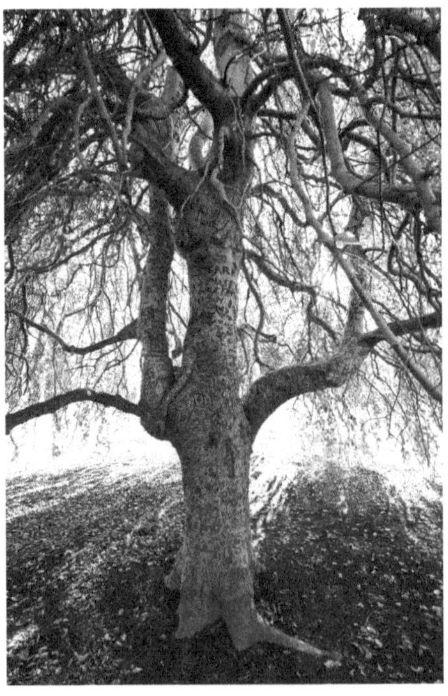

It is imperative for professionals to emphasize the countless strengths occurring in teens' and young adults' lives. When working with young people in therapy, identifying inner, family, and community strengths serves as a touch point for further therapeutic exploration. These strengths may then be built upon to literally form the foundation of an adolescent's or young adult's life. Strengths identification during these life stages may influence whether or not a person attends college, college choice, selection of a major, career planning, mate preference, and other salient life decisions. Formulation of positive, forward-thinking action plans may develop as a result of collaborative identification of assets, gifts, and strengths in an individual's life.

Strengths themselves serve as a vital component of treatment. By identifying and building upon individuals' unique assets and strengths at this point in their lives, a positive framework for their further development may be explored. Look toward their inner gifts, family supports, friendships (past and present), abilities, desire for change, as well as community-based opportunities and assets. Cultural beliefs, spirituality, and religious values and beliefs can also be built on to solidify a foundation for growth and healthy development. Recognition of these gifts and strengths serves as a springboard for change by facilitating growth and promoting self-discovery.

Although strengths-based practice involves focusing on the positive aspects of individuals' lives and building on these, by no means should problems be minimized or remain unheard. Instead, a shift is made to focus on how one has coped or managed while living with any given problem or challenge. Lessons learned from this process may be emphasized as well in order to facilitate growth (Sharry, Madden, & Darmody, 2003). Recognition of life's injustices, such as discriminatory practices and oppression, must also be factored into the equation. These factors, however, may be viewed on a screen of resilience.

When working with individuals who have suffered traumatic events in their young lives such as rape or sexual abuse, remain cognizant that clients should be encouraged to express painful emotions surrounding these events. They should be allowed to tell their stories in a compassionate, caring, and safe environment. Clients' reactions to such traumatic events may be viewed through a strengths lens as well. For instance, instead of viewing clients' responses such as dissociation or acting-out behaviorally as negative maladjustment, professionals may choose to see these as reactions to difficult circumstances. Examining how clients have coped with severe traumas using a strengths focus can promote a sense of freedom in the therapeutic process. Nonproductive responses may be reframed as survival mechanisms that people may now move beyond through personal growth and healing. Additional strength, insight, and capabilities may be gained, allowing teens or young adults to more effectively cope with past, present, and future hurdles in their lives (Wade, 1997).

A basic tenet of the strengths perspective is that everyone has strengths, although they may not be apparent at first glance. Part of this perspective involves an understanding that clients approaching practitioners already have valuable information about their own situations. According to Dennis Saleebey, who has written extensively regarding the strengths perspective, "clients come into view when you assume that they know something, have learned lessons from experience, have hopes, have interests, and can do some things masterfully. These may be obscured by the stresses of the moment, submerged under the weight of crisis, oppression, or illness but, nonetheless, they abide" (2002, p. 14). It is essential for the therapist to assist teens and young adults in finding, identifying, and naming their strengths throughout the assessment and treatment process. It is partially through practitioners' faith and belief in clients' abilities and potential that young people will begin to have faith and believe in themselves.

For those mental health practitioners who have concerns about using strengths as a focus of their assessments, interventions, and treatments, the following perspective may be advantageous in their transition process. Sharry, Madden, and Darmody feel that, "As therapists, it can be difficult to focus on a client's strengths, particularly if we are having difficulties in working with a case, are pessimistic about the possibility of progress, or feel negative about the client. However, this is often the best time to think differently and to begin to view the client and the therapy through a strengths based lens" (Sharry, Madden, & Darmody, 2003, p. 8). Though this transition process from problem-based to strengths-based practice may place some individuals outside of their comfort zones, many will eventually discover that these changes will result in positive outcomes for many of their clients.

One solution-focused way of viewing strengths identification is by how therapists and clients collaboratively "identify qualities that clients can realistically bring to bear on the problem situation" (Walsh, 2007, p. 106). This process involves building on and developing innate traits that already exist within the client or within the context of the clients' social relationships. The process, in and of itself, can be therapeutic, as well as serving as a context for finding solutions to problems.

When practitioners respond to the needs of clients, the strengths approach tends to examine many of the assets that clients already possess. By utilizing a strengths approach, even brief, time-limited interventions have an increased chance of success, as clients are building on skills, gifts, family, and community foundations that have already been laid. At times, the strengths perspective may focus on the future, while identifying and employing obscured strengths. This type of practice orientation may contribute to the reduction in emotions related to feeling helpless and hopeless. This may be because clients feel that if someone else in a position of power believes they have potential and strengths, they may feel that they have value as well (Johnson & Yanca, 2004). While past problems or dysfunctions should not be minimized, they do not necessarily need to be the sole focus of intervention.

In addition, the figurative and literal communities in which adolescents and young adults learn, socialize, interact, and grow affect their current and future development. Community asset assessments may be conducted with the young person to assist in mapping out locations, literal and virtual, that may serve to improve, enhance, or alter his or her own life. By playing an active role in this mapping, he or she may more clearly identify with potential pathways toward change, progress, and growth. Furthermore, encouragement from adult members of the community, such as members of the clergy, teachers, friends of the family, and those who have overcome adversity, may promote the fostering of resilience in youth and young people.

Resiliency is a term frequently heard in relation to the strengths perspective and positive psychology. Resiliency focuses on the application of individuals' gifts, assets, and strengths toward the amelioration of challenges and overcoming of obstacles in their lives (Kirst-Ashman, 2011). Although people may have made less than favorable decisions in the past, in many instances they will actually have ideas or suggestions about what would help them in the future (Saleebey, 2002). Questions in this book promote resilience through facilitating "coping" or "handling" even the most challenging, extremely difficult, or overwhelming situations. Pertinent activities also promote assisting individuals with identifying their own unique skill-sets and strengths.

One way resilience is commonly explained to clients and students is as an ability to "bounce back" from stressful events. This can be further illustrated in a concrete manner through the use of simile when comparing a person to different types of rock. The practitioner may explain that a person is like a rock. For example, if sandstone is dropped onto a cement driveway, it is likely to shatter, or at a minimum, fracture. In contrast, granite, a much stronger type of rock, is more likely to remain whole and intact when dropped onto the same type of cement driveway. The goal is to attempt to make people remain whole or restore them to an intact state, like the granite, in the face of hardship.

Another example that could be used to examine this point would be the comparison between wax and diamonds. When placed near a normal or typical flame, wax is likely to melt whereas diamonds will retain their original shape. Instead of melting when faced with the fires of life, people need supports to withstand these flames in order to restore or retain their intact selves. To reiterate, by identifying and building upon individuals' strengths, resilience can be fostered to buffer against the adversities of life.

Strengths can be integrated into the therapeutic storytelling process with adolescents and young adults. Storytelling itself serves as a medium for self-disclosure and assists in identification of resources, intelligences, assets, and strengths. In the context of therapy, it is recommended that practitioners "Listen to clients' stories instead of zipping through an assessment protocol. Stories and narratives often contain within their plots and characterizations evidence of strengths, interests, hopes, and visions" (Saleebey, 2002, p. 88). Furthermore, when applying the strengths approach to storytelling, "the therapists may incorporate their positive attitudes into storytelling by selecting the positive features about the major and minor characters in the stories. If positive features cannot be found, create them. Therapists may also envision how the characters can be further developed" (Slivinske & Slivinske, 2011, p. 21).

Strengths Based-Questions

Questions designed to elicit strengths from characters within the provided stories, and eventually from each individual client, are included within the activity sheets that accompany each story. Examples of strengths-based questions incorporated throughout the activities in this text are as follows:

- What could this person do to feel better?
- How does this person deal with or how could this person deal with his or her feelings?
- How does this person cope with being so quiet?

- How did she end up getting help to handle the stress of possibly being pregnant?
- How was she able to handle the situation?
- Why are this person's friends and family concerned about him?
- What did you do to cope emotionally with the situation?
- What did you learn from the situation?
- What did the person do to help him or her to make this difficult decision?
- Who can the girl in this story turn to for help?
- How can this girl cope in a positive way with the stress she is experiencing?
- Who did you turn to for help regarding what happened?
- What are your strengths that can help you to cope with your situation?
- What are some good things about you and your parents?
- What could this person do to feel better and to cope with the situation?
- How did you or could you cope with the break up in a positive way?
- What are some of your own strengths, not related to the relationship?
- What are some healthy choices you could make?
- What positive steps could you take to make your life better?
- What are five good qualities that you have?
- How could this person cope with the mental or physical pain he or she is experiencing?

Other more generalized questions regarding strengths may be integrated into discourse with clients. Suggestions for asking strengths-based questions when working with teenagers and young adults include the following:

- What are you good at doing?
- What activities or hobbies do you enjoy?
- What do you really like about yourself as a person?
- How would your closest friends describe you?
- What are your favorite books and movies?
- What are some strengths or positive traits about yourself?
- What are some positive aspects of your relationship with your mother?
- What are some positive aspects of your relationship with your father?
- What are some good things about your relationship with your friends?
- What are some positive aspects about your relationship with your boyfriend or girlfriend?
- Who do you know that you can really count on to be there for you in your life?
- What are your favorite subjects in school?
- In what areas do you excel academically?
- What hobbies do you enjoy the most and why?

Other types of strengths-based questions that hold significant relevance to those at the brink of adulthood include what Saleebey would call "Possibility Questions." These are especially significant during the teen and young adulthood years, as individuals are in the process of becoming and formulating who they will be, and what they will do, for life. Examples of a few of these types of questions follow:

- "What are your hopes, visions, and aspirations?"
- "What are your special talents and abilities?"
- "What fantasies and dreams have given you special hope and guidance?" (Saleebey, 2002, p. 89)

At times, mental health practitioners' may benefit from asking themselves questions based in positive psychology that are directed toward their work with their own clients. This self-reflection and self-assessment of practice remains vital toward incorporating current, fresh, and insightful ideas into interactions with clients. The following strengths-oriented questions proposed by Sharry, Madden, and Darmody (2003) and designed for therapists' self-inquiry remain relevant to resourceful and insightful practice:

- "What strengths does this impasse reveal about your work as a therapist?"
- "What is going well in your work with this client or in his or her contact with professional services? What has gone well in the past?"
- "What are you doing constructively as a therapist in spite of any difficulties or the current impasse?"
- "What resources and strengths do you have as a therapist that might be helpful to this client?" (p. 91).

Strengths-Based Statements

Strengths-based, affirmative statements or phrases may also be integrated into discussions with clients when appropriate. The statement may then be followed up on by examining how these positive traits, strengths, and relationship assets may be applied to aspects of their personal, academic, and professional lives. At this point in their lives, it is particularly salient to identify and apply strengths toward personal and career aspirations. Examples of these types of statements or phrases follow:

- I have noticed you are really talented in mathematics. Careers in teaching, engineering, and computer science might be options for you.
- I can tell you really enjoy writing, and you seem to excel in that area. You might consider being an editor, author, or teacher.
- It seems that your best friend always seems to be there to support you when you need her. You are lucky to have her in your life.
- You seem to really be taking good care of yourself physically. You are eating right and not drinking too much alcohol. You should be proud of that.

- You are very athletic. You might want to consider careers that involve some aspect of athletics, since you like it so much.
- Your family must care about you a lot. You seem to be able to count on them, and even though they don't have a lot of money, it is nice that they are helping you to pay for your books for college.
- You are very sociable and get invited to a lot of parties. You must be popular. That would help you in a job in sales.
- You are dependable, trustworthy, and reliable. Those are all excellent qualities that people look for in an employee and a spouse.
- You have great potential to improve in that area. Just don't give up and keep on trying. You can succeed.
- You are a stronger person than you think. Even though all of these bad things have happened to you, you keep on trying and you have not given up. You are still around, even though many of your friends are not. I know that all of this is hard to handle, but I think you can get through it.

PLAN Method of Intervention

We also suggest utilizing the PLAN method as a tool when working with, advising, or treating adolescents and young adults. The PLAN method of intervention provides concrete steps and actions that can be taken to formulate goals, action plans, and build upon strengths. When using the PLAN method, the following steps can be applied to treatment of individuals' personalized challenges and strengths. The PLAN method of intervention is explained below:

Positive action creates positive lifestyles.
Look to the future.
Activate your strengths, both inside and out.
Never give up on yourself.

When using this method, first elaborate on each of the core concepts in the PLAN method with clients. Modify facets or details of the method as needed to meet the needs of individual clients. Chapter 18, Strengths, contains activity sheets that may be accessed on the accompanying website when discussing these suggested modalities.

Positive Action

When discussing positive action with teens and young adults, it would be appropriate to ask them what they are doing in their lives, and if necessary, how they can change what they are doing in a positive way. The idea being that positive action plans will lead to positive and healthy changes in their lives, in turn, ultimately creating positive lifestyles.

Practitioners, when assisting clients in this manner, may help clients identify what they need to do in order to achieve positive outcomes or results in their lives.

For example, if a young adult who is slightly depressed completes a college application and is accepted into a university, this would be the first step, or positive action. Hopefully, the next step would be positive change. Perhaps if he studies, is busy using the university athletic facilities, and meets new friends, his positive change might be that his mood improves because of engagement in positive activities. Ideally, after awhile, as his actions become like second nature, he will develop a more positive lifestyle overall, which is step three in the process. In some instances, his mood may be lifted naturally as part of the progressive cycle of change.

Look to the Future

Looking to the future involves trying to assist teens and young adults, some of whom may have a "present orientation" that does not involve forward thinking, to envision possibilities and opportunities in their forthcoming lives. This may entail examining what they would like to be doing or engaged in a week from now, a month from now, six months from now, a year from now, and so on. Simple goal setting and action plans may enable individuals who are "stuck" to move forward and progress in their lives. Individuals, with help from friends, family members, and professionals, may contemplate and compare and contrast who they feel they are now, versus who they are in the process of becoming.

Activate Your Strengths

First, positive traits, attributes, strengths, and resources of the individual must be identified. Ways in which a person can then transform those abstractions into verifiable actions, thoughts, and behavioral changes may be discussed in the therapeutic setting. Practitioners may ask a client, "What are you doing?" or "What can you do to make that strength come alive for you?" Actual application of strengths in real life situations will ideally occur. Identifying positive qualities and strengths in youth and young adults enables potential pathways to be paved toward change and development of possible solutions to be found to challenging life situations.

Connections between strengths and career choice may be recognized. If a person excels in mathematics, perhaps practitioners could discuss careers in which mathematics is utilized, such as teaching, higher education, research, engineering, architecture, business, manufacturing, computer science, and the like. Visits, conversations, connections or emails with people employed in those fields could be arranged. Job shadowing may be an option. These would be examples of ways in which strengths could potentially be activated.

This is almost akin to the concept of transferable skills in career development. For example, if a young person is gifted at musical performance but is currently unsure about what direction her life will follow regarding career ambitions, a practitioner may be helpful in sorting out realistic available options. Discussion may ensue regarding possible college majors, such as music performance or teaching. Careers not requiring degrees, such as performance, may be discussed, and so forth. Pursuing music as an avocation instead of a vocation may also be explored. The hope is that valuable insight will be gained, allowing the young person to decide whether and how she desires to integrate particular strengths into her life.

Never Give Up on Yourself

It is not uncommon for young people in treatment to feel discouraged, confused, or depressed. They may feel that one or two life mistakes or a few poor decisions cannot be overcome. They may need reassurance that they can succeed if they continue to try, without giving up on themselves. If relationships fail, they need to be reminded that new ones may begin. If they do not succeed in a particular major in college, they may need instruction and encouragement that perhaps that area was not their strength, but if they persevere they will find a subject in which they excel. If they do not give up on themselves, they can find something positive, whether in careers or relationships, that works for them. With help from caring professionals, unearthing of obscured talents, assets, gifts, and strengths may transpire.

Additional Resources

Bertolino, B. (2010). *Strengths-based engagement and practice: Creating effective helping relationships.* Upper Saddle River, NJ: Pearson.

Helton, L. R., & Smith, M. K. (2004). *Mental health practice with children and youth: A strengths and well-being model.* Binghamton, NY: Haworth Social Work Practice Press.

Saleebey, D. (2013). *The strengths perspective in social work practice* (6th ed.). Upper Saddle River, NJ: Pearson.

Slivinske, J., & Slivinske, L. (2011). *Storytelling and other activities for children in therapy.* Hoboken, NJ: John Wiley & Sons.

6

Social Adjustment and Peer Acceptance

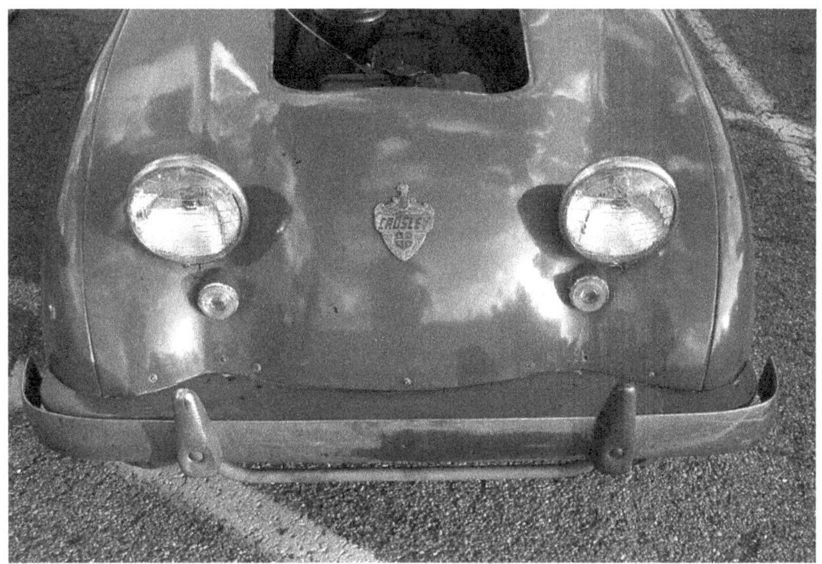

Key Practice Issues and Story Selection

Many adolescents and young adults will struggle with experiences dealing with attempting to "fit in" or be accepted by members of their peer group. Some may need assistance learning social skills that have not been mastered during middle childhood. Others may just need their self-esteem or confidence boosted during this sometimes challenging and confusing period of life.

Teens tend to be very influenced by friends, and during adolescence it becomes increasingly significant to belong to a specific peer group. This is usually the small cluster of friends that they relate with on a day-to-day basis, and who may positively or negatively influence the teens' thoughts and actions. In addition, teens may have a special affiliation with a larger group of peers based on memberships in clubs, interests, hobbies, athletics, academics, or acting-out behaviors (Newman & Newman, 2012).

Many may reflect on their own personal experiences as a teenager or young adult and recall fondly the "group" that they were closest with emotionally. In the United States, this special group of peers typically may attend parties together, go to football games on Friday nights, and sit together with one another at lunch. Regarding special affiliations, members of this group may also be a part of a larger social context. They may see each other and others at band practice, soccer practice, or speech team practice. These social relationships are an important part of the growing up process in our society.

However, others may recall the pain and frustration apparent when these positive, healthy social interactions are lacking. They may reflect upon what it was like to sit all alone at the lunch table day after day, feeling isolated and lonely, like an outcast. Memories may exist of lonely nights at home listening to depressing music, peers not asking them to parties, and not having dates on Friday or Saturday nights.

In reality, many people encounter both the positive and negative experiences associated with belonging or not belonging to a particular peer group. Emotions associated with these events fall along a continuum of feeling completely alone and like a social outcast to feeling like the most popular person in the school. When appropriate and beneficial to the adolescent client, practitioners may choose to share their own adolescent and young adult experiences that contributed to their maturation as a human being. These may help to normalize adolescents' and young adults' own typical development struggles of the day.

Suggestions for practitioners to help adolescents and young adults to improve their self-esteem, social skills, and valuable relationships include:

- Model appropriate social interactions, with the intent that the client will emulate the therapist and imitate positive social interactions.
- Conduct interactive role plays with the client, allowing him or her to practice actual social interactions in a nonthreatening environment.
- Teach individuals how to overcome typical difficulties such as disagreements in both friendships and romantic relationships.
- Teach teenagers and young adults' positive self-care when faced with negative relationship interactions that sometimes occur.
  - Examples of self-care include:
    - Eating healthy foods such as fruits and vegetables
    - Engaging in exercise such as biking or walking
    - Meditating or participating in yoga to aid in relaxation and stress relief
    - Writing in a journal
    - Listening to mood-enhancing or soothing music
    - Drawing or painting to express one's self
    - Participating in an activity that is particularly enjoyed

The story "I'm Not a Loser" was chosen for inclusion in this book because it exemplifies the feelings of not fitting in that many teens will experience. The client may identify with the main character, and social skills can be further explored based on the client's individual needs. Strengths can be further developed too, such as the ability to maintain a friendship.

"She Doesn't Even Notice Me" demonstrates the difficulties encountered by an adolescent boy who likes a classmate but is unsure of himself, not knowing how to approach her romantically. Many people will undoubtedly relate to this all too common scenario. The practitioner and client can discuss appropriate and positive ways of interacting, and role plays may be performed to allow for practice and development of social skills.

In the story "I'm Kind of Quiet," a person wants to reach out to others, but is unsure regarding how to accomplish this. The character experiences anxiety as displayed through sweating and not knowing what to say or how to act with others. Again, the use of role plays that demonstrate how to interact in a friendly, appropriate manner may be beneficial, as well as teaching clients relaxation techniques such as guided imagery and controlled breathing as an adjunct to this story.

Additional Resources

Covey, S. (2004). *The 7 habits of highly effective teens personal workbook.* New York: Fireside.

Foa, E. B., & Andrews, L. W. (2006). *If your adolescent has an anxiety disorder: An essential resource for parents.* New York: Oxford University Press.

Geldard, D. (2009). Promoting self-care behaviors. In K. Geldard (Ed.), *Practical interventions for young people at risk* (pp. 13–21). London, UK: Sage.

Shannon, J. (2012). *The shyness & social anxiety workbook for teens: CBT and ACT skills to help you build social confidence.* Oakland, CA: New Harbinger Publications, Inc.

I'm Not a Loser

I don't fit in here... and I probably never will. I simply can't stand it here. I am so different than all of them. I don't like the things that they like, and I guess they can sense it. This is just who I am—I can't help that. They don't have to be so rude to me though. They all could treat me with some respect—not like I'm some kind of useless freak with two heads that vomits fire and ashes. I mean, what the hell—they could make me feel a little bit more included couldn't they?

Really, how many parties have I been invited to since I've been here? One, and that's just because of my friend Josh. I suppose one friend is better than no friends. If I didn't know him, people probably wouldn't even speak to me because they think I'm such a loser. Well, they don't know me very well, because I am not a loser. I am not going to eat dirt anymore. I am really going to show them and I will prove to them I am not a loser. I will tell you what I am going to do, but only if you promise not to tell anyone else.

Instructions: Tell, write, or draw the answers to the following questions.

I'm Not a Loser Questions: Level 1

1. How is this person feeling?
2. Why does this person feel this way?
3. What could this person do to feel better?
4. How could this person make friends?
5. How would you finish this story?

I'm Not a Loser Questions: Level 2

1. Do you know anyone who has ever felt like the character in this story?
2. Can you tell me what it is like for him or her to feel this way?
3. What does he or she do when he or she feels this way?
4. How does this person deal with or how could this person deal with his or her feelings?
5. What is his or her story?
6. How would you change his or her story if you could?

I'm Not a Loser Questions: Level 3

1. Have you ever felt like the character in the story?
2. Can you tell me what it is like for you when you feel badly?
3. What could you do to try to feel better?
4. How could you make some new friends?
5. What is your story?
6. How would you change your story if you could?

My Story: Level 4

Instructions: Tell, write, or draw your own story.

She Doesn't Even Notice Me

I see her once in awhile in the hallway at school. Her name is Sierra, and she is simply beautiful, with flowing dark silky hair and kind, deep brown pools of dark chocolate for eyes with soft, tender, smooth, creamy skin. I know her skin is soft because our hands touched once when she dropped her pencil and I picked it up for her. She sits two seats over in my English class, and once in awhile she glances my way and smiles. It gives me chills all over when she does that. For the most part though, she doesn't even seem to notice me.

I would really like to get to know her better, but I don't really know how to do that. I am way too nervous to go up and talk to her. There is no way I could do that. I wouldn't even know what to say. Maybe I could ask her friend for her cell number, and then I could text her—but she might think that's creepy. Maybe I should ask her for her cell number, or I know, I could "friend" her on the Internet. But what if she doesn't "friend" me back? Okay, I'm really stressing out here now. I've got to get to know this girl better, but how!

Instructions: Tell, write, or draw the answers to the following questions.

She Doesn't Even Notice Me Questions: Level 1

1. How is this person feeling?
2. Why does this person feel this way?
3. How could this person get to know Sierra better?
4. How could this person overcome his anxiety and nervousness when it comes to girls?
5. How would you finish this story?

She Doesn't Even Notice Me Questions: Level 2

1. Do you know anyone who has ever felt like the character in this story?
2. Can you tell me what it is like for him or her to feel this way?
3. What does he or she do when he or she feels this way?
4. How does this person deal with or how could this person deal with his or her feelings?
5. What is his or her story?
6. How would you change his or her story if you could?

She Doesn't Even Notice Me Questions: Level 3

1. Have you ever felt like the character in the story?
2. Can you tell me what it is like for you when you like someone?
3. What could you say or do to try to get to know someone better?
4. What is your story?
5. How would you change your story if you could?

My Story: Level 4

Instructions: Tell, write, or draw your own story.

I'm Kind of Quiet

My mother says she worries about me because I'm so quiet. Well, maybe I just don't like to talk to that many people. They make me nervous, you know? It is hard for me to carry on a conversation with other people sometimes. I just don't know what to say, so I start to stumble over my words and sometimes I even start to sweat because I get so nervous.

I do have one good friend that I've known forever. I do get lonely sometimes though. I suppose it would be nice to have a few more guys to hang out with, but I'm not really sure how to go about doing that. I wouldn't mind meeting a nice girl either, but I get really nervous when I have to talk to girls that I like.

Instructions: Tell, write, or draw the answers to the following questions.

I'm Kind of Quiet Questions: Level 1

1. Why is this person so quiet?
2. How does being quiet help or hurt him?
3. How could this person feel more comfortable talking with others?
4. What could this person say or do to make more friends?
5. How would you finish this story?

I'm Kind of Quiet Questions: Level 2

1. Do you know anyone who is very quiet?
2. Can you tell me what it is like for him or her to be so quiet?
3. What could this person do to learn better social skills?
4. How does this person cope with being so quiet?
5. What is his or her story?
6. How would you change his or her story if you could?

I'm Kind of Quiet Questions: Level 3

1. Are you ever quiet like the character in the story?
2. Can you tell me what it is like for you when you are quiet? How does it feel?
3. What could you say or do to try to get to know someone better?
4. What is your story?
5. How would you change your story if you could?

My Story: Level 4

Instructions: Tell, write, or draw your own story.

7

Sexuality

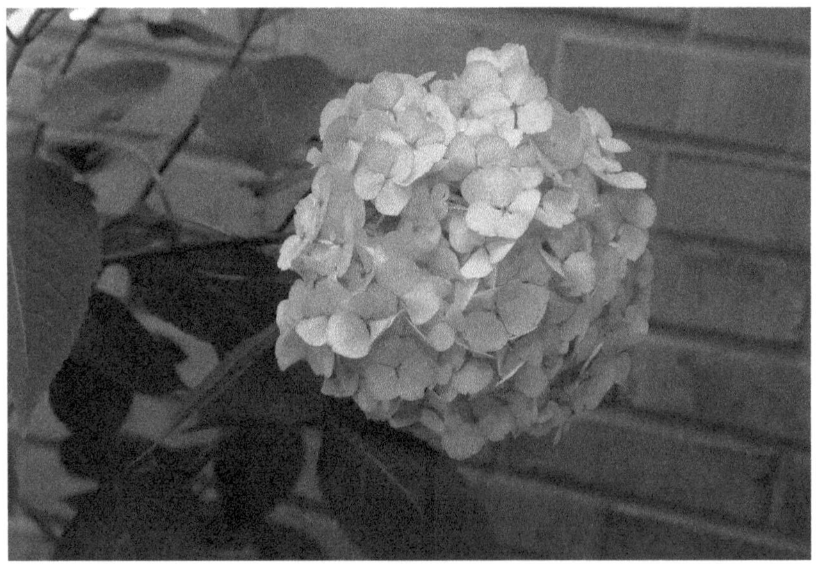

Key Practice Issues and Story Selection

For many, adolescence is a time of curiosity and exploration regarding relationships and sexuality. This period in teens' and young adults' lives may be fascinating and exciting while simultaneously bewildering and confusing. Many may experiment with different aspects of intimacy and sexuality in an effort to find connectedness. Others may act-out sexually in an effort to gain attention or as a reaction to stressful or negative life events.

It is quite common and typical for developing adolescents to experience numerous biological changes. In females, adjusting to alterations in hormonal levels may be challenging or perplexing. Young males may at times be uncomfortable with experiencing sexual arousal at unwanted times. However, both boys and girls are likely to encounter an enhanced libido. Because of the shifts in their hormonal states, both young men and young women will experience increased emotionality, which may frustrate parents and adolescents alike (Shriver, Byer, Shainberg, & Galliano, 2002).

Challenges regarding sexuality during this time in life include break-ups with boyfriends or girlfriends, poor communication between partners regarding expectations, conflicts associated with moral beliefs, and unplanned pregnancies. These important life-changing events may alter teens' and young adults' perceptions of themselves temporarily, and in some circumstances, permanently. In some instances, teens and young adults may become pregnant and prepare for the duties and responsibilities associated with parenting at a young age.

When teenagers and young adults who are not equipped or prepared to raise children become pregnant and parent their children, they may be confronted with extra difficulties and experience losses. Many in their age group may not have the skills to cope with the unique challenges of young parenthood that emerge, even though the young parents may be loving and responsible and care for their children very much. According to Shriver, Byer, Shainberg, and Galliano, some potential consequences of having children early include:

- Loss of fulfillment of dreams due to childcare and work responsibilities.
- Lack of full development of the young person's potential, especially for adolescent girls and young women.
- Due to early responsibilities, teenage males and young men may forgo attending college in order to work and provide for their child or family.
- Grandparents may help with childcare, although they are preparing for enjoying retirement.
- Teenage males may be unprepared to parent and may not be involved in their children's lives.
- Young parents in general may be less prepared emotionally, behaviorally, and financially to raise children (2002).

In addition, when other high-risk behaviors such as consuming alcohol and taking drugs are thrown into the sometimes tumultuous mix of adolescence, unplanned sexual relations may occur. This at times may leave individuals feeling embarrassed and confused. When intoxicated, teens and young adults may be even less concerned with protection from sexually transmitted diseases and pregnancy.

The media, including television and the Internet, now afford adolescents and young adults easy access to sexually graphic material, which has the potential to affect their sexual beliefs and development. The long-term effect of viewing this material is inconclusive. However, television and other media tend to be a major source of information regarding sexuality for those in adolescence, and many times portrayals of sexuality are distorted and unhealthy (Hyde & DeLamater, 2006).

Tips to help young people struggling with sexuality during adolescence and young adulthood include:

- Encourage them to share their fears or confusion with a caring adult or therapist.
- Reassure them that they are normal for feeling unsure or confused regarding sexual issues.
- Facilitate conversations surrounding exploration of their own values and beliefs regarding their own sexual thoughts and behaviors.
- Encourage them to discuss and delineate any possible positive or negative consequences associated with engaging in specific types of sexual behaviors.
- Explore with them concerns or questions regarding birth control, dependent upon their own and their family's religious beliefs and values.
- Discuss issues related to and answer questions regarding transmission of sexually transmitted diseases.
- Facilitate conversations about the effects of alcohol, drug use and abuse, as well as its affect on judgment related to sexual decision making abilities.

The story, "I Think I'm Pregnant," addresses the emotional and complicated matter of a teenage girl who suspects she is pregnant after missing her menstrual period. She then has no support from her boyfriend and is fearful of telling her parents about the pregnancy concerns because of their disapproval. Those who have been in this situation are likely to identify with the stress experienced by the young woman in the story. It also may be used to facilitate conversations regarding physical and emotional consequences of sexual expression among those who are considering becoming sexually active.

"How Could I Have Been So Stupid?" is a story in which a teenager or young woman feels betrayed and used by a young man who she believed loved her. People in this situation need care and support while recovering from this type of emotional hurt. Practitioners should discuss warning signs to be aware of that could potentially signal harmful relationships. Possible ways to avoid these negative relationship pitfalls could be investigated.

Adolescents and young adults are likely to experience many questions and concerns regarding their own sexuality. One such concern is addressed in the stories "How Do I Know If I'm Ready" and "Am I Ready?" in which young people are unsure about when a relationship should progress to a more intimate level. This subject may be examined with the therapist in the context of individuals' and families' unique and personalized belief systems. Physical and emotional ramifications of sexual activity and expression, both positive and negative, may be discussed by using these stories as springboards. Responsible relationships and sexuality may also be explored.

The vignette titled "Drunk" delves into the relationship between negative consequences and risks of alcohol and drug use when experiencing emotional confusion. Individuals who relate to this story may then examine, through the eyes of another, the dangers of risky behavior involving sexuality, drugs, and alcohol. We hope that insights will be gained and healthy, positive coping mechanisms may be learned.

Additional Resources

Freitas, D. (2008). *Sex and the soul: Juggling sexuality, spirituality, romance, and religion on America's college campuses.* New York: Oxford University Press.

Gordon, P. A., Tschopp, M. K., & Feldman, D. (2004). Addressing issues of sexuality with adolescents with disabilities. *Child and Adolescent Social Work Journal*, 21(5), 513–527.

Russell, S. T. (2005). Conceptualizing positive adolescent sexuality development. *Sexuality Research and Social Policy*, 2(3), 4–12.

Somers, C. L., & Paulson, S. E. (2000). Students' perceptions of parent-adolescent closeness and communication about sexuality: Relations with sexual knowledge, attitudes, and behaviors. *Journal of Adolescence*, 23(5), 629–644. doi: http://dx.doi.org/10.1006/jado.2000.0340.

I Think I'm Pregnant

I can't believe it. I don't know what I'm going to do or who I can turn to. I told my best friend yesterday that I missed my period. I am usually really regular—but now I am ten days late. My mom and dad are going to kill me. They don't even know I have a boyfriend, and they definitely don't know I'm having sex.

It gets worse too. I told my boyfriend I am pregnant yesterday, and he wants nothing to do with me. I love him and don't know what I am going to do without him. He just walked away from me in school like nothing had happened. What am I going to do? At least my best friend is there for me.

Instructions: Tell, write, or draw the answers to the following questions.

I Think I'm Pregnant Questions: Level 1

1. Who can the girl in this story turn to for help?
2. Why is she so upset?
3. How can this girl cope in a positive way with the stress of possibly being pregnant?
4. How would you finish this story?

I Think I'm Pregnant Questions: Level 2

1. Do you know a girl who ever thought she was pregnant?
2. Who did she talk to about possibly being pregnant?
3. How did she end up getting help to handle the stress of possibly being pregnant?
4. How was she able to handle the situation?
5. What is her story?
6. How would you change her story if you could?

I Think I'm Pregnant Questions: Level 3

1. Do you think that you might be pregnant?
2. What is it like for you thinking you might be pregnant?
3. Who can you turn to for help regarding your possible pregnancy?
4. What are your strengths that can help you to cope with maybe being pregnant?
5. What is your story?
6. How would you change your story if you could?

My Story: Level 4

Instructions: Tell, write, or draw your own story.

How Could I Have Been So Stupid?

He used me…How could I have been so stupid? I know we only dated for a few months, but he told me he loved me, and I believed him. Now he's gone. I slept with him and he left me. He texted me yesterday and told me that he doesn't want to see me anymore.

I really trusted him and believed him when he said he loved me, but I don't think he cared about me at all. I feel so hurt and angry all at the same time. He's such a jerk. My friends even warned me about him, but I didn't listen to them. How am I supposed to deal with all of this stuff happening to me?

Instructions: Tell, write, or draw the answers to the following questions.

How Could I Have Been So Stupid Questions: Level 1

1. Who can the person in this story turn to for help?
2. Why is the person so upset?
3. How can this person cope in a positive way with what has happened?
4. How would you finish this story?

How Could I Have Been So Stupid Questions: Level 2

1. Do you know a person who has felt used?
2. How did he or she feel emotionally?
3. What did he or she do to cope emotionally with the situation?
4. What did he or she learn from the situation?
5. What is his or her story?
6. How would you change his or her story if you could?

How Could I Have Been So Stupid Questions: Level 3

1. Have you ever felt used?
2. How did you feel emotionally?
3. What did you do to cope emotionally with the situation?
4. What did you learn from the situation?
5. What is your story?
6. How would you change your story if you could?

My Story: Level 4

Instructions: Tell, write, or draw your own story.

How Do I Know if I'm Ready?

I've been dating Marissa for five months now, and I really like her. In fact, I think that I'm in love with her and that she might be the one. Besides that, she is absolutely beautiful and I can hardly hold it together when I'm around her. When we kiss, it's just so great—like we are on another planet together or floating in outer space. I can't really even explain how awesome it is. I just want to kiss her forever.... But I think I want and need more from her.

I have told her that I want to go further, and she thinks she wants to too, but how do we know if we are ready to go to the next level? And then there's the problem of birth control—what should we use if we do? Should I get something or should she? It all seems very unromantic—but I don't want to get her pregnant; we are still in school.

Instructions: Tell, write, or draw the answers to the following questions.

How Do I Know if I'm Ready Questions: Level 1

1. What is this boy so concerned about?
2. What else is he feeling?
3. What could he do to help him make this difficult decision?
4. What are the pros and cons of becoming sexually active?
5. How would you finish this story?

How Do I Know if I'm Ready Questions: Level 2

1. Do you know anyone who has ever felt like the character in this story?
2. Can you tell me what it is like for him or her to feel this way?
3. What did the person do to help him or her make this difficult decision?
4. What were the pros or cons of this person's decisions regarding being sexually active?
5. What is his or her story?
6. How would you change his or her story if you could?

How Do I Know if I'm Ready Questions: Level 3

1. Have you ever felt like the character in this story?
2. Can you tell me what it is like for you to feel this way?
3. What could you do to help you make this difficult decision?
4. What are the pros or cons of your decisions regarding being sexually active?
5. What is your story?
6. How would you change your story if you could?

My Story: Level 4

Instructions: Tell, write, or draw your own story.

Am I Ready?

My boyfriend and I have been dating for a really long time now, and he says he'd like to take our relationship to the next level—you know, by having sex. How do I know if I'm ready? I really like him and I think I love him, but it seems like such a big deal. Then there's the pregnancy thing. What if I get pregnant? I'm way too young for that. This is all so confusing for me.

He said he'll wait for me until I'm ready—but he's ready now, and I want to make him happy. What am I going to do? How do I make this important decision?

Instructions: Tell, write, or draw the answers to the following questions.

Am I Ready Questions: Level 1

1. What is this girl so concerned about?
2. What else is this person feeling?
3. What could she do to help her make this difficult decision?
4. What are the pros and cons of becoming sexually active?
5. How would you finish this story?

Am I Ready Questions: Level 2

1. Do you know anyone who has ever felt like the character in this story?
2. Can you tell me what it is like for him or her to feel this way?
3. What did the person do to help him or her make this difficult decision?
4. What were the pros or cons of this person's decisions regarding being sexually active?
5. What is his or her story?
6. How would you change his or her story if you could?

Am I Ready Questions: Level 3

1. Have you ever felt like the character in this story?
2. Can you tell me what it is like for you to feel this way?
3. What could you do to help you make this difficult decision?
4. What are the pros or cons of your decisions regarding being sexually active?
5. What is your story?
6. How would you change your story if you could?

My Story: Level 4

Instructions: Tell, write, or draw your own story.

Drunk

I went out last night when I was really upset about what happened. I probably shouldn't have gone. At the club, I started drinking drink after drink, just to forget about it. Then before I knew it I was really drunk. I smoked a little pot too, and then I was really out of it. I just wanted to forget everything, and before I really realized what I was doing, I was getting into this guy's car and going home with him. Well, you can pretty well imagine the rest of what happened...

Instructions: Tell, write, or draw the answers to the following questions.

Drunk Questions: Level 1

1. How is this person feeling and why?
2. Why did the person get drunk and high?
3. What do you think the person did after getting into the car with the guy?
4. What are the risks involved with getting drunk or high and getting into a car with someone?
5. How would you finish this story?

Drunk Questions: Level 2

1. Do you know anyone who has ever felt like the character in this story?
2. Can you tell me what it is like for him or her to feel this way?
3. What did the person learn from his or her experience?
4. What is his or her story?
5. How would you change his or her story if you could?

Drunk Questions: Level 3

1. Have you ever felt like the character in this story?
2. Can you tell me what it is like for you to feel this way?
3. What did you learn from your experience?
4. What is your story?
5. How would you change your story if you could?

My Story: Level 4

Instructions: Tell, write, or draw your own story.

My Sexuality Questions

Instructions: Tell, write, or draw the answers to the following questions.

1. What are your values and beliefs about sexuality and becoming sexually active with someone?
2. How long do you feel you should know someone before becoming sexually active?
3. Should you be married before becoming sexually active?
4. Do you feel you are emotionally prepared enough and mature enough to become sexually active with a particular person?
5. What are some possible positive and negative consequences of becoming sexually active?

Personal Choices

1. Tell, write, or draw about some positive aspects of birth control.
2. Tell, write, or draw about some negative aspects of birth control.
3. Will you or do you choose to use birth control? Why or why not?

8

Abuse, Sexual Assault, and Exploitation

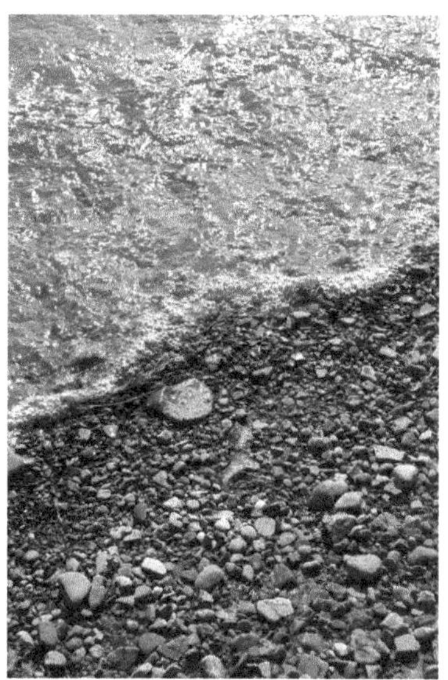

Key Practice Issues and Story Selection

Unfortunately, for many young adolescents, particularly young female teenagers, their first sexual experience may occur as a result of abuse, assault, or exploitation. Thus, in many instances for young females, their first sexual experiences are not planned or desired (Newman & Newman, 2012). Of course, this may be the case for young adolescent boys as well, although it tends to be less well-documented. Boys in general are less likely to report sexual abuse or rape. According to the Centers for Disease Control, nationally in the United States 9.3% of African American teens, 7.8% of Hispanic teens, and 6.9% of white teens of high school age had been raped (Centers for Disease Control, 2008).

Those who have experienced sexual assault or abuse may experience detrimental effects from the ensuing trauma. Some possible deleterious outcomes include substance abuse, depression, anxiety, post-traumatic stress reactions, lack of trust in relationships, anger issues, delinquency, and so forth. Males or females who were abused by someone of the same-sex may experience concerns or confusion regarding their sexual identity. When assisting victims of abuse or assault it is imperative to provide sincere emotional support and to assure victims that they are not at fault (Coleman & Farris-Dufrene, 1996).

During the course of the development of the therapeutic relationship, abusive experiences may also be discussed from childhood and adolescence, even if the client is currently an adult. Other emotionally difficult times may also be recalled. Some solution-focused methods that concentrate on strengths-oriented questioning to promote growth may be valuable to this type of circumstance. The following questions posited by Sharry, Madden, and Darmody may be used with clients as they overcome adversity and search for positive people, environments, and qualities that enabled them to survive very difficult times (2003).

- "If you could change what happened to you, what would you change?"
- "How did you cope with these experiences?"
- "Who in your family supported you through these times?"
- "Who outside your family supported you?"
- "If you feel these experiences left you with a negative "script" or legacy, how would you like to change it?"
- "What have you learned or would you like to learn from this experience?" (p. 53)

These types of questions fit particularly well with therapeutic storytelling techniques, as in a sense they are permitting or allowing a client who has experienced trauma to rewrite or rescript his or her own personal narrative. Thus, hypothetical mastery and control over one's life and environment, in a figurative sense, could be gained. This could allow for greater or enhanced feelings of empowerment for those who have been disempowered.

Additional suggestions for helping victims of rape or sexual abuse include:

- Discuss all sensitive issues in a private location to protect the dignity of clients.
- Listen attentively to victims' emotions and concerns regarding the assault or abuse.
- Avoid inadvertently blaming the victim for the assault or abuse.
- Offer emotional support.
- Advocate for victims' rights if the court system and the police are involved in the situation.
- Serve as a liaison for victims attempting to negotiate the stress of police interviews and the court system.
- Teach effective coping techniques for handling intense emotions surrounding the abuse or rape, including anger management.

Those who have been raped may experience a wide range of emotions, including feelings of helplessness and a lack of control. In addition, they may feel angry, depressed, or anxious. Many individuals who have been raped will experience rape trauma syndrome and may exhibit and experience symptoms related to their traumatic experience. Some of these symptoms include:

- Disorganization Phase: A person feels frightful, angry, and in denial that the rape has occurred. She or he may question how she or he could have avoided the assault, and may blame herself or himself.
- Controlled Reaction Phase: A person in this phase may appear calmer and less emotional, although she or he is still seriously harmed from the assault.
- Reorganization Phase: A person adjusts to reintegrating her or his life and adjusting to living from day-to-day after the rape (Matsakis, 2003). Issues that are salient to the rape survivor during this phase include:
  - Gaining a sense of feeling safe
  - Overcoming feelings of fear
  - Dealing with the feelings of loss (such as losing trust in others)
  - Redeveloping a personal identity (Matsakis, 2003).

Events from the past such as child sexual abuse or rape may continue to burden adolescents and young adults. This may still sometimes occur even if a person has successfully coped with the traumatic effects of the assault. The vignette, "A Long Time Ago," successfully addresses these issues. It portrays a person who is still sometimes upset regarding negative aspects of the past. This individual is acknowledging this very real pain but also successfully copes with it in a positive manner. This story is beneficial for further exploring strengths-based coping mechanisms with teens and young adults.

In the story "An Older Guy Likes Me," an adolescent experiences confusion and does not know what to do regarding a troubling circumstance in which an older man is trying to take advantage of her sexually. This story could be utilized with adolescents who have been abused or exploited by someone older than them. They may relate to and identify with the character in the story, and may feel less alone in their emotional challenges. A safe, supportive environment allowing for emotional expression may contribute to healing. Conversations related to ways to prevent future exploitation would also be beneficial.

As mentioned previously, sexual assault and rape are more common than many believe. In the story "Raped," the emotional trauma in the aftermath of a sexual assault is presented through the female character in the story. Many will relate to this story, and it may help those who have been assaulted by allowing them a means to express their own story of trauma. Comfort, support, and hope for future healing could be provided in a safe and caring environment.

Additional Resources

Briere, J. N., & Lanktree, C. B. (2012). *Treating complex trauma in adolescents and young adults*. Thousand Oaks, CA: Sage.

Foa, E. B., & Andrews, L. W. (2006). *If your adolescent has an anxiety disorder: An essential resource for parents*. New York: Oxford University Press.

Mason, S. E., & Clemans, S. E. (2008). Participatory research for rape survivor groups: A model for practice. *Affilia: Journal of Women and Social Work*, 23(1), 66–76. doi: 10.1177/0886109907310459

Rothbaum, B. O., & Foa, E. B. (1999). *Reclaiming your life after rape: Client workbook*. New York: Oxford University Press.

Willis, D. G. (2009). Male-on-male rape of an adult man: A case review and implications for interventions. *Journal of the American Psychiatric Nurses Association*, 14(6), 454–461. doi: 10.1177/1078390308326518

A Long Time Ago

It happened so long ago, but sometimes, deep down, it really still bothers me. Sometimes, it still hurts. I wish it had never happened or that I could just make it go away. But it did happen and I can't make it go away. But I can tell you what I can do. I can live well and I can take care of myself. I am a good person and I deserve to be treated well. I deserve to be respected for the smart, kind, and nice person that I am. I won't let anyone mistreat me, not if I can help it. I will be an example for others that a person can experience bad things but still have a wonderful life. In fact, I think I'm going to go call a friend and invite her out for lunch. Then maybe we'll go walking on the trail in the park for a little bit to take my mind off of things. I am sure that would make me smile, and before I know it I'll be in a good mood again!

Instructions: Tell, write, or draw the answers to the following questions.

A Long Time Ago Questions: Level 1

1. Why do you think this person is bothered by his or her past?
2. How is this person coping with what has happened in the past?
3. How else could he or she cope?
4. How would you finish this story?

A Long Time Ago Questions: Level 2

1. Do you know anyone who is bothered by his or her past?
2. How is this person coping with what has happened in the past?
3. How else could this person cope?
4. How was he or she able to cope with what happened?
5. What is this person's story?
6. How would you change his or her story if you could?

A Long Time Ago Questions: Level 3

1. Have you ever felt upset because of something that happened in the past?
2. How did you feel?
3. How did you cope with what happened in the past?
4. What are your strengths that can help you to further cope with your situation?
5. What is your story?
6. How would you change your story if you could?

My Story: Level 4

Instructions: Tell, write, or draw your own story.

An Older Guy Likes Me

I really don't know what to do—I actually feel pretty confused. I'm only fourteen and this older guy keeps hitting on me. I met him online and we've been texting a lot. He is thirty-five and has a girlfriend that he lives with. I really like him though, and I've been telling him all of my problems and how depressed I've been lately. He is such a good listener and he makes me feel really special. He tells me how pretty I am all of the time. He even texted me and said he loves me. I think I love him.

I really want to run away to be with him but he says that other people wouldn't understand our special kind of love. Maybe he's right—after all he is older than me. He probably knows best. He has a good job and his own place too. He's so handsome and mature.

Then the other day he said that if he's going to listen to all of my problems and be there for me all of the time that we should have sex—or he's not going to hang out with me or text me anymore. I've never even kissed a boy before! I told my best friend about him and she thinks I should stay away from him—but I told her he is everything to me and I love him. I can't imagine my life without him. What should I do? I need some good advice.

Instructions: Tell, write, or draw the answers to the following questions.

An Older Guy Likes Me Questions: Level 1

1. Who can the girl in this story turn to for help?
2. Why is she so upset?
3. How can this girl cope in a positive way with the stress she is experiencing?
4. How would you finish this story?

An Older Guy Likes Me Questions: Level 2

1. Do you know anyone who thought she was in love with an older guy?
2. Who did she talk to about the older guy?
3. What did she end up doing?
4. How was she able to handle the situation?
5. What is her story?
6. How would you change her story if you could?

An Older Guy Likes Me Questions: Level 3

1. Has an older guy ever come on to you?
2. How did you feel when that happened?
3. Who can you turn to for help regarding your situation with this older guy?
4. What are your strengths that can help you cope with your situation?
5. What is your story?
6. How would you change your story if you could?

My Story: Level 4

Instructions: Tell, write, or draw your own story.

Raped

I feel like in an hour's time my whole life has been changed—because it has been. Last night I was walking home after practice and I was approached by a guy who seemed nice enough—but then he grabbed me and pulled me into the woods. Then he raped me... I feel so horrible, like I just can't believe it happened. I froze and couldn't move when it happened because I was so scared. It almost seems unreal. It was terrifying...

He told me that if I told anyone he would kill me, and that he knows where I live. What am I supposed to do now? I feel like I will never be the same person that I was... How will I recover from this?

Instructions: Tell, write, or draw the answers to the following questions.

Raped Questions: Level 1

1. Who can the girl in this story turn to for help?
2. Why is she so upset?
3. How can this girl cope with what has happened to her?
4. How would you finish this story?

Raped Questions: Level 2

1. Do you know anyone who has been raped?
2. Who did she turn to for help?
3. What did she end up doing?
4. How was she able to cope with what happened to her?
5. What is her story?
6. How would you change her story if you could?

Raped Questions: Level 3

1. Have you ever been raped or sexually assaulted?
2. How did you feel when that happened?
3. Who did you turn to for help regarding what happened?
4. What are your strengths that can help you to cope with your situation?
5. What is your story?
6. How would you change your story if you could?

My Story: Level 4

Instructions: Tell, write, or draw your own story.

9

Parents

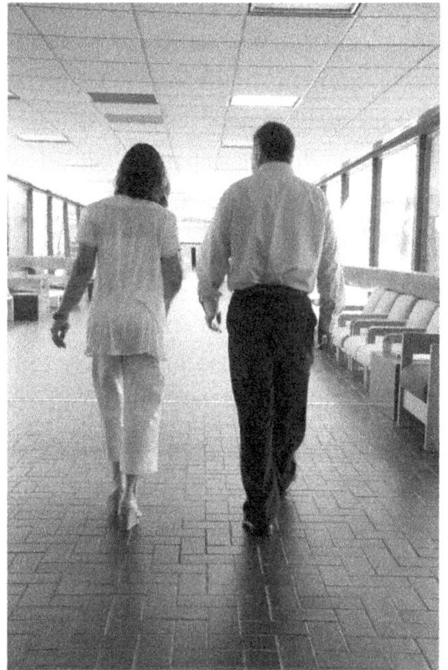

Key Practice Areas and Story Selection

Parents play an integral part in the continuing development and progression from adolescence into adulthood. Inevitably, as adolescents break away from their parents in an effort to establish their own unique identities, conflicts may arise between many parents and teenagers. With many individuals now living at home with their parents for longer periods, these conflicts may also extend well into young adulthood. This may contribute to increased friction in the home and potential for confusion of roles and responsibilities regarding household chores and financial issues.

Typical parent-adolescent conflicts are likely to center around individuation of the adolescent. Individuals may attempt to maintain more privacy than their parents are willing to give or accept. Parents, in turn, may attempt to protect their children by controlling their actions and behaviors, but this may be adamantly opposed by some adolescents. Although adolescents may resist parental limit setting, enforcement of age-appropriate limits is vital. Many adolescents will actually, at some level, crave this type of parental attention and interpret it as a sign of parental caring, love, and concern.

However, in the age of cell phones and Internet technology, it is increasingly difficult for parents to monitor and control their adolescents' actions and interactions. Parents may feel distressed about inappropriate or dangerous interactions with strangers, acquaintances, and friends. These concerns are warranted, as some teens and young adults are now engaged in activities such as "sexting," or the practice of sending nude pictures of themselves or others via mobile phones. In addition, many teens and young adults have almost constant access to video cameras and can instantaneously post lewd, inappropriate, and lamentable moments to the Internet. Inevitably, many will later regret postings or videos made in a moment of poor judgment.

Many adolescents and young adults have parents who are in the process of becoming divorced or are divorced. This is a particularly frustrating time for all involved. Families navigate through the pain of lost relationships, feelings of inadequacy, divided loyalties, and lowered incomes. Adolescents and young adults who experience this also are more likely to feel anxious, feel depressed, engage in antisocial behavior, have health problems, and perform less well in school. They are also more likely to be less committed in their relationships and to divorce as adults. Developmentally, the family unit that is charged with socializing our youth cannot operate as well when it becomes dysfunctional and dissolves (Clark-Stewart & Dunn, 2006; Harvey & Fine, 2010). Meeting with a therapist may assist these individuals overcome these obstacles and find ways to more effectively mature and develop.

Adolescents and young adults who have had one or both parents incarcerated often experience increased levels of emotional and behavioral problems. They may become withdrawn, have attention deficit problems, develop maladaptive coping mechanisms, act out, become more aggressive, have poor school performance, become delinquent, have poor socialization, and the like. Often they are exposed to additional risk factors such as abuse, neglect, and poverty among others. Additionally, they may suffer the shame and social stigma of a parent's incarceration. The factors mentioned earlier often negatively affect their development, including the ability to organize their behavior toward the achievement of future goals, delay gratification, and become independent and self-sufficient. Finally, such individuals have poorer treatment outcomes than those adolescents and young adults who do not have a parent in jail (Gabel & Johnston, 1995; Phillips, et al. 2002). These youth need the opportunity to tell their stories and be heard.

Suggestions for parents and adolescents encountering relationship changes or conflicts include:

- Try to respect one another as individuals.
- Give appropriate degree of privacy and freedom to adolescents as long as trust has not been seriously violated.
- Remain involved in the teenager's or young adult's life. They may need parental advice and guidance more than their parents realize.
- Converse openly with and listen to teens and young adults, even if parents disagree intellectually, spiritually, or morally with what they have to say.
- Invite adolescents or young adults to participate in enjoyable activities that the family unit engaged in when they were younger children. This may help parents stay connected to their loved ones.
- Encourage teens or young adults to involve parents in some of their new and developing interests in life.

The desire for a teen to have more freedom and privacy is exemplified in the story "My Dad's Such a Jerk." Some adolescents may identify with the feelings experienced by a teenager when a father is attempting to protect his child. From the perspective of the teen however, this behavior is viewed as intrusive. This type of story could benefit teens and their families by exploring, with professionals, to find the right balance between the need for adolescent protection and autonomy.

Conflict between an adolescent and a mother is demonstrated through the vignette "Leave Me Alone." Typical disagreements regarding commonplace activities of daily life such as performing household chores are portrayed. The adolescent also believes that his or her parent does not realize what it is like to be a teenager. This story could open the door for healthy and honest communication between parents and their teenage children.

Family turmoil and feelings of hurt and rejection are examined in the story "The Divorce." Children often know that their parents have been arguing and often blame themselves for the impending separation and divorce. The negative emotions experienced by adolescents and young adults merit exploration. This story may aid those who are experiencing this type of situation to work through these negative emotions, determine that they are not the cause of the divorce, and learn positive ways to effectively adjust and cope with their new circumstances.

The consequences associated with the incarceration of a parent are dealt with in the story "My Dad's in Jail." Adolescents and young adults are old enough to know that their parents disappointed them and their family. They may still love their parents, but their respect for them has diminished. This story may enable those who are familiar with this situation to discuss their feelings, express desires for life circumstances to be different, and assist them in developing constructive coping mechanisms.

Additional Resources

Kerig, P. K., Schulz, M. S., & Hauser, S. T. (Eds.). (2012). *Adolescence and beyond: Family processes and development*. New York: Oxford University Press.

McGoldrick, M., & Hardy, K. V. (Eds.). (2008). *Re-visioning family therapy: Race, culture, and gender in clinical practice* (2nd ed.). New York: Guilford Press.

Miller, S. B. (2012). *When parents have problems: A book for teens and older children who have a disturbed or difficult parent* (2nd ed.). Springfield, IL: Charles C. Thomas Publisher, Ltd.

Sachs, B. (2013). *Family-centered treatment with struggling young adults: A clinician's guide to the transition from adolescence to autonomy*. New York: Routledge.

My Dad's Such a Jerk

My dad's such a jerk. He always just tells me what to do. I think he wants to totally control my life. These are the things I can't stand about him: he goes into my room all of the time without knocking on the door, he tries to read my online conversations with my friends, and he even takes my cell phone and checks my texts all of the time. He doesn't know it, but I just delete the ones I don't want him to see. Anyway, he doesn't really understand the things we are texting about anyway because we text in code.

He says he is just trying to look out for me, but I feel like he is looking over my shoulder all of the time. I have no privacy! I need my space! How can I let him know that I am not some five year old kid anymore? In a few years, I won't even be living at home. I can't wait until I am eighteen and an adult so I can do whatever I want whenever I want!

Instructions: Tell, write, or draw the answers to the following questions.

My Dad's Such a Jerk Questions: Level 1

1. Why does the person in this story think his or her dad is a jerk?
2. Why is he or she so upset?
3. Why do you think this person's father is checking up on him or her?
4. What can this person do to improve his or her relationship with his or her father?
5. How would you finish this story?
6. How would you change this story if you could?

My Dad's Such a Jerk Questions: Level 2

1. Do you know anyone who doesn't get along with his or her parents?
2. Why don't they get along?
3. How could this person improve his or her relationship with his or her parents?
4. How would you finish his or her story?
5. How would you change his or her story if you could?

My Dad's Such a Jerk Questions: Level 3

1. Do you get along with your mom or dad?
2. What are some things you would like to change in your relationship with your parents?
3. How could you improve your relationship with your parents?
4. What are some good things about you and your parents?
5. What is your story?
6. How would you change your story if you could?

My Story: Level 4

Instructions: Tell, write, or draw your own story.

Leave Me Alone

My mom's always on my back about something! Why doesn't she just leave me alone. She nags me about picking up my room, and she says I text my friends and boyfriend way too much. What does she know anyway, she's just old and cranky.

She probably doesn't even remember what it was like to be a teenager!

Instructions: Tell, write, or draw the answers to the following questions.

Leave Me Alone Questions: Level 1

1. Why is the girl in this story upset with her mother?
2. Why do you think her mother acts the way she does?
3. What can this girl do to improve her relationship with her mother?
4. Do you think her mother remembers what it was like to be a teenager?
5. How would you finish this story?
6. How would you change her story if you could?

Leave Me Alone Questions: Level 2

1. Do you know anyone who doesn't get along with his or her parents?
2. Why don't they get along?
3. How could this person improve his or her relationship with his or her parents?
4. How would you finish his or her story?
5. How would you change his or her story if you could?

Leave Me Alone Questions: Level 3

1. Do you get along with your mom or dad?
2. What are some things you would like to change in your relationship with your parents?
3. How could you improve your relationship with your parents?
4. What are some good things about you and your parents?
5. What is your story?
6. How would you change your story if you could?

My Story: Level 4

Instructions: Tell, write, or draw your own story.

The Divorce

We all knew something was terribly wrong when our parents got us out of bed in the middle of the night. Mom and Dad had a terrible fight earlier this evening, just like the many fights they have had before. My older sister warned me that this day was coming, but I didn't believe her. My younger brother just stood there and cried because he was so upset and scared. They told us they were getting divorced and that we had to pick with whom we wanted to live. Before I could answer, my older sister gave me "the look," which told me to keep my mouth shut as she knew what I was thinking. She knew I was mad at both of them for ruining our family and that I didn't want to live with either of them anymore. I just wanted this horrible night to go away. We kept wondering what we did wrong.

Instructions: Tell, write, or draw the answers to the following questions.

The Divorce Questions: Level 1

1. Why is this person so upset?
2. What do you think is happening in this family?
3. What can this person do to cope with his or her parents' divorce?
4. How would you finish this story?
5. How would you change this story if you could?

The Divorce Questions: Level 2

1. Do you know anyone who has been upset over his or her parents' divorce?
2. Why is he or she upset?
3. How could this person cope with his or her parents' divorce?
4. How would you finish his or her story?
5. How would you change his or her story if you could?

The Divorce Questions: Level 3

1. Have you ever felt upset over your parents' divorce?
2. Why were you upset?
3. How could you cope with your parents' divorce?
4. What are some good things about you and your parents?
5. What is your story?
6. How would you change your story if you could?

My Story: Level 4

Instructions: Tell, write, or draw your own story.

My Dad's in Jail

I love my dad, and I really miss him. He used to take me out to eat on Saturdays when he had enough money. I liked hanging out with him. He really did try to get it together. He had been doing so much better not using and he had even quit drinking. I was so proud of him. But then he let me down, and he messed up in a huge way. What he did was so bad that now he's in jail. Now I visit him once in awhile in jail. I still love him, and I wish he was out. I know he loves me too. It's hard to go to the jail though because I have to talk to him on the phone through the glass. It feels so uncomfortable for me. I just wish things were different.

Instructions: Tell, write, or draw the answers to the following questions.

My Dad's in Jail Questions: Level 1

1. How does the person in this story feel about his or her dad being in jail?
2. What issues are bothering him or her?
3. Why do you think his or her father is in jail?
4. What can this person do to improve his or her relationship with his or her father?
5. How would you finish this story?
6. How would you change the story if you could?

My Dad's in Jail Questions: Level 2

1. Do you know anyone who has a parent who is in jail?
2. What issues bother this person?
3. How could this person improve his or her relationship with his or her parent?
4. How would you finish his or her story?
5. How would you change his or her story if you could?

My Dad's in Jail Questions: Level 3

1. Is your mom or dad in jail?
2. What issues bother you about your relationship with your mom or dad?
3. How could you improve your relationship with your mom or dad?
4. What are some good things about you and your parents?
5. What is your story?
6. How would you change your story if you could?

My Story: Level 4

Instructions: Tell, write, or draw your own story.

10

Relationships

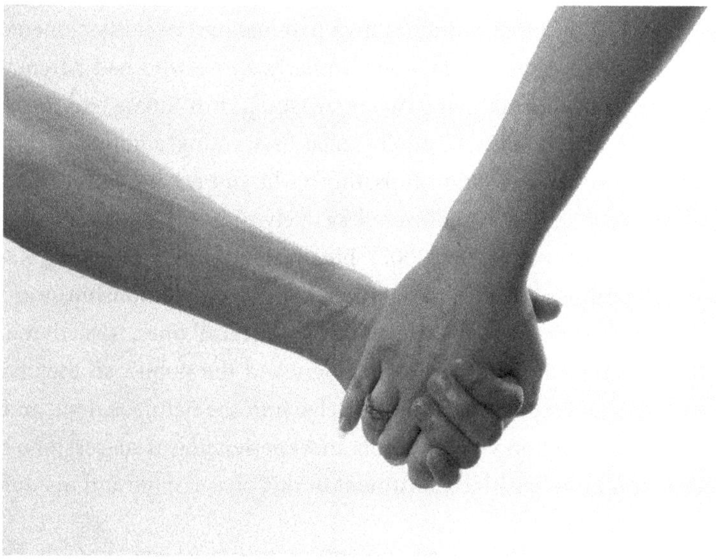

Key Practice Issues and Story Selection

Relationship issues and forming one's identity are key concepts central to developing into a healthy teenager and young adult. Issues surrounding conflicts within dating relationships and friendships abound during these phases of life. It is not uncommon for adolescents and young adults to experiment with and "try on" different types of dating relationships, as well as a variety of friendship groups or circles. Some people will be a "good fit," while other relationships wither and dissolve. These are all typical developmental steps and tasks in the formation of a solid identity that move a person further toward the development of intimacy in friendship and romantic relationships.

The importance of positive and satisfying relationships during adolescence and young adulthood cannot be overstated, as they have been found to be associated with increased emotional, cognitive, and social abilities. Individuals who experience such relationships are more likely to become independent, productive adults. The skills learned in social relationships assist youth in enhancing their social functioning at home, in school, and the workplace. When families, friends, or others in the environment do not provide positive support systems, impaired development and its related deficiencies often result (Ashford & LeCroy, 2011; Milevsky, 2011). For example, poor parental and peer relationships have been found to be associated with having fewer friends, higher levels of depression and drug use, and lower grade point averages (Field, Diego, & Sanders, 2002). Likewise, those without individuals to act as mentors were found to have more unexcused absences from school and poorer scholastic competence (Rhodes, Grossman, & Resch, 2000). Also, youth whose relationships with parents were described as being distant often reported worse adjustment at school (Wainright, Russell, & Patterson, 2004). Likewise, Ma and Huebner (2008) found that more negative parental and peer attachments were associated with lower levels of life satisfaction. Similarly, those who had parental relationships that were described as not being caring, trusting, or intimate had greater difficulty forming positive attachments in adolescence and young adulthood (Fraley & Davis, 1997). Regarding romantic relationships, those who did not have healthy, romantic relationships at the end of high school were less likely to marry and to cohabitate in early adulthood (Raley, Crissey & Muller, 2007). Finally, regarding race, Wang, Kao, and Joyner (2006) found that those involved in interracial, romantic relationships were more likely to terminate them earlier than those involved in intraracial ones. Also, they are less likely to reveal these relationships to family members and the public, so they had less social support. Therefore, therapists must always delve into the nature, extent, and types of relationships that adolescents and young adults are experiencing as successful relationships are associated with more positive adjustment in this phase of life and in adulthood whereas unsuccessful ones are not.

Positive friendships can buffer adolescents through difficult times and serve as a protective factor. It is typical for adolescents to spend much more time with peers than with parents during this life stage. Adolescents who have learned to develop and maintain positive friendships tend to sustain a more positive outlook on life and to be better adjusted emotionally (Levine & Munsch, 2011).

Tips to encourage positive relationship skills in adolescence include:

- Modeling and role playing how to compromise within the context of friendships and romantic relationships.
- Encouraging the development of negotiation skills.
- Exploring sensitivity issues related to the wants and needs of others to promote strong, healthy relationships (Levine & Munsch, 2011).

- Recommending that adolescents join clubs or sports groups in which they have a particular interest in order to develop friendships or romantic relationships with those who hold similar interests.

The heartbreaks of adolescence and young adulthood are portrayed through the scenario "My Boyfriend Broke Up with Me," in which a young woman is saddened by the break up between her and her boyfriend. Many adolescents and young adults will identify with this common situation. With the help of family, friends, and professionals, positive methods of coping with these typical developmental challenges may be learned.

"Confused…" addresses the bewilderment sometimes experienced by those attempting to establish a firm identity in life but who become lost in the process of individuation. Decisions may feel overwhelming to some individuals, and it is not uncommon to experience stress regarding who to date, who to have as friends, where to attend college, what career to choose, and so forth. With the help of a concerned professional, a person encountering such dilemmas may benefit from sessions that involve clarifying and setting current and future manageable life and relationship goals.

In the scenario "Heartsick," a young woman is so consumed with her boyfriend that she does not want to spend any time away from him. She is upset that he has interests besides her, and she is jealous that he is spending time with friends. If someone identifies with this type of all-consuming, infatigable, possessive relationship, they may benefit from discussing appropriate and healthy relationship boundaries, as well as exploring his or her own identity, including likes and dislikes, goals, aspirations, and interests.

Additional Resources

Eastham, C. (2011). *The truth about dating, love & just being friends.* Nashville, TN: Thomas Nelson.

Fox, A. (2005). *The teen survival guide to dating & relating: Real world advice on guys, girls, growing up, and getting along.* Minneapolis, MN: Free Spirit.

Rogers, V. (2010). *Let's talk relationships: Activities for exploring love, sex, friendship, and family with young people.* London, UK: Jessica Kingsley Publishing.

Woodward, L. J., Fergusson, D. M., & Horwood, L. J. (2002). Romantic relationships of young people with childhood and adolescent onset antisocial behavior problems. *Journal of Abnormal Child Psychology, 30*(3), 231–243.

My Boyfriend Broke Up with Me

I feel so heartbroken. I can't believe we broke up. I didn't want to break up, but Dakota wanted to date other girls. I really thought that we would be together forever, and that he loved me. He was my first real boyfriend. Now I feel like I will never find someone to love me the way that Dakota loved me.

He made me feel so special and he's just such a great guy. He's so funny and nice and always makes me smile. He said we could still be friends, but I don't want to just be friends. I want so much more than that because I'm still in love with him.

I thought we were going to get married after we both went to the same college together. Then I thought we would get an apartment together and just be so happy. Now that will never happen, and I'll never find someone as great as Dakota!

Instructions: Tell, write, or draw the answers to the following questions.

My Boyfriend Broke Up with Me Questions: Level 1

1. Why is this person so upset?
2. What else is this person feeling?
3. What could this person do to feel better and to cope with the situation?
4. What does this person want out of her life?
5. How would you finish this story?

My Boyfriend Broke Up with Me Questions: Level 2

1. Do you know anyone who has ever had a girlfriend or boyfriend break up with him or her?
2. What did he or she feel like when this happened?
3. What does this person do when he or she feels this way?
4. How does this person deal with or how could this person deal with his or her feelings?
5. What is his or her story?
6. How would you change his or her story if you could?

My Boyfriend Broke Up with Me Questions: Level 3

1. Have you ever been through a bad break-up with a boyfriend or girlfriend?
2. Can you tell me what it was like for you when your boyfriend or girlfriend broke up with you?
3. How does this make you feel?
4. How did you or could you cope with the break up in a positive way?
5. What is your story?
6. How would you change your story if you could?

My Story: Level 4

Instructions: Tell, write, or draw your own story.

Confused...

Sometimes I just get so confused...There are so many choices and decisions to make right now in my life! I have to decide who to hang out with, who my real friends are, who to date, and everything else. It just seems so overwhelming! Besides all of this I am supposed to decide what I want to do with the rest of my life! Right...like, I have no idea really.

By the way, what am I supposed to do with my life? Should I go to college? Should I get a job? Should I move? Now you see what I mean—I have no idea what to do with my life. I wish someone would just tell me what to do; then maybe I wouldn't have to decide for myself!

Instructions: Tell, write, or draw the answers to the following questions.

Confused Questions: Level 1

1. Why is this person feeling so confused?
2. What are the choices that this person is worried about making?
3. What could this person do to make these choices in a positive way?
4. What does this person want out of his or her life?
5. How would you finish this story?

Confused Questions: Level 2

1. Do you know anyone who has ever felt confused about his or her life?
2. What are the choices that this person is worried about making?
3. What could this person do to make these choices in a positive way?
4. What does this person want out of his or her life?
5. How would you finish his or her story?
6. How would you change his or her story if you could?

Confused Questions: Level 3

1. Do you ever feel very confused in your own life?
2. Can you tell me what it is like to feel so confused and overwhelmed?
3. What are the choices you are worried about making?
4. What could you do to make these choices in a positive way?
5. What do you want out of your life?
6. How would you finish your story?
7. How would you change your story if you could?

My Story: Level 4

Instructions: Tell, write, or draw your own story.

Heartsick

I feel sick today. I just don't want to do anything. My body's not sick though—I'm heartsick. I miss Braden so much and I just want to be with him all of the time. I just can't stop thinking about him. It's like I have Braden on the brain. I don't understand why I can't be with him.

I know I will see him tomorrow. He's coming over my house and we are going to catch a movie. I just don't get why he had to go out with his friends tonight without me. What's that all about? I thought he loved me. He does love me, I think . . .

Well, at least I get to see him tomorrow. I think I will text him now to see how his night is going.

Instructions: Tell, write, or draw the answers to the following questions.

Heartsick Questions: Level 1

1. How is the girl in this story feeling?
2. Is it okay for Braden to go out with his friends without her?
3. What could this person do to make herself feel better when Braden is busy?
4. What are some characteristics of a healthy relationship?
5. How would you finish this story?

Heartsick Questions: Level 2

1. Do you know anyone who has ever felt sad or lonely when he or she missed a girlfriend or boyfriend?
2. What did this person do to make him or herself feel better about missing a girlfriend or boyfriend?
3. What did this person do to make healthy relationship choices?
4. How would you finish his or her story?
5. How would you change his or her story if you could?

Heartsick Questions: Level 3

1. Have you ever felt sad or lonely when you missed your boyfriend or girlfriend?
2. Can you tell me what it is like for you feeling so sad and lonely?
3. What could you do to feel better about missing your boyfriend or girlfriend?
4. What are some of the positive and negative things about your current relationship?
5. What are some of your own strengths, not related to the relationship?
6. How would you finish your story?
7. How would you change your story if you could?

My Story: Level 4

Instructions: Tell, write, or draw your own story.

11

Eating Issues

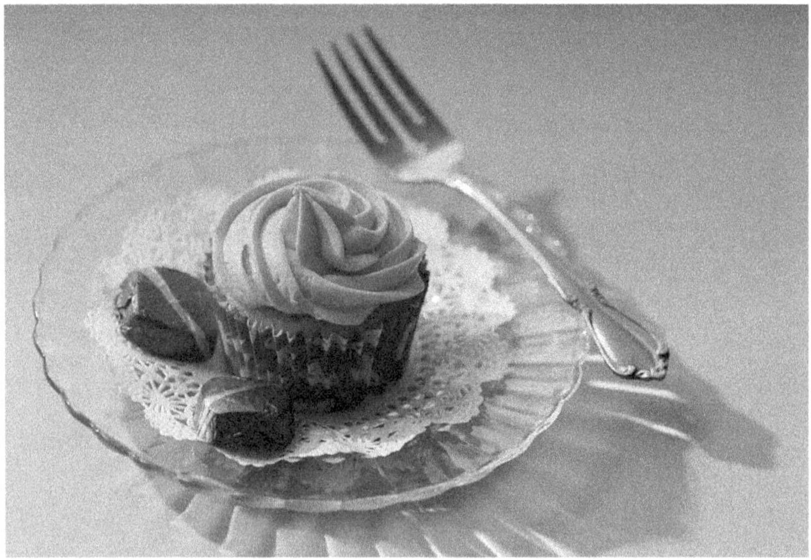

Key Practice Issues and Story Selection

During adolescence and young adulthood, young men and women are at risk for encountering physical and mental health problems surrounding weight, diet, and nutritional issues. Negative health consequences may occur as a result of either over eating, binge eating, dieting excessively, or binging and vomiting or using laxatives. All of these place an individual at risk for developing illnesses, diseases, and for suffering emotional and social consequences based on these maladaptive behaviors.

Being overweight is a concern of many adolescents and young adults. Between the 1980s and the year 2000, the rate of obesity for adolescents in the United States almost tripled. This gain leads to an increased risk of adolescents and young adults of developing type 2 diabetes (Ashford & LeCroy, 2010). In addition, other health problems may arise in the future, including arthritis, heart disease, stroke, and vulnerabilities to certain cancers. Many believe that eating "fast food," unhealthy snacks, and consuming larger portions has contributed to this dilemma. Lack of significant exercise is another contributing factor.

Besides the very real physical problems that can result from being obese or overweight, a variety of social problems may occur as well. At any age, a social stigma may be attached to being overweight. This can be particularly difficult to handle during adolescence, when peer acceptance and the further development of a self-concept are simultaneously occurring (Ashford & LeCroy, 2010). Rejection by peers and lowered self-confidence are possibilities that may transpire due to being overweight. In adolescence, and in young adulthood, many individuals struggle with relationship issues, including the challenge of finding the right person to date. This challenging issue may become even more complicated for some if they perceive that they are being rejected based on physical appearance issues related to weight.

Another issue frequently occurring during adolescence and young adulthood is anorexia, which is characterized by excessive weight loss, refusal of many foods, obsessive exercise, and feeling that one is overweight, even though one is well below a healthy weight. This condition is sometimes life threatening. Those with bulimia tend to binge eat, and then vomit or abuse laxatives to avoid gaining weight (Newman & Newman, 2006).

Some girls may feel pressure to be thin based on perceptions seen in the media and popular culture. This potentially may influence some teenagers and young adults to imitate this behavior in an attempt to be perfect or accepted, which theoretically may contribute to eating disorders in some girls and young women. However, other factors may contribute to eating disorders among girls as well as boys, such as low self-esteem. Factors that may affect self-esteem, particularly of girls, include "issues of attachment, of family bonds, of grief, of lack of self-knowledge during traumatic adolescence, of physiological change, of brain development, of hormone cycles" (Gurian, 2002, p. 20), and so forth. These life challenges affect boys as well, and both genders are also impacted by stressors in the family such as divorce and parents who are so busy that it is difficult for them to spend the time to be there for teens and young adults (Gurian, 2002).

Some suggestions to help teens with problems resulting in binge or addictive eating include:

- Recommend that individuals keep a food log in which they track what they have eaten during a particular day.
- Encourage people to write about how they feel emotionally and physically before and after eating certain foods and binge eating.
- Brainstorm with teens and young adults regarding the motivations behind their eating behaviors, and attempt to formulate a plan for replacing the negative eating behaviors with positive alternative behaviors such as:
  - Journaling
  - Calling or texting a friend

- Walking
- Exercising
- Meditating

Developing a positive lifestyle in adolescence or young adulthood lays the foundation of health for life. "Healthy," portrays a young person proactively attempting to address concerns regarding healthy living. This story could be used with many individuals who actively attempt to lead lives oriented toward wellness, and it may serve as a model for those struggling with integrating positive decisions into their lives. In addition, the vignette depicts the use of exercise and lifestyle choices as a method of constructive coping.

In the story "I Think I'm Fat" the character believes that he or she is extremely overweight, when in fact, the character is likely anorexic. This story could be used with clients to allow for expression of deep feelings regarding one's body image. Cognitive distortions could be elucidated and challenged in order to facilitate healthy change and self-acceptance. This scenario may be used as a supplemental form of expression for a person who has an eating disorder, or who is at risk for developing an eating disorder, in addition to other relevant treatment modalities based on the practitioner's own professional philosophy and training.

The story "I'm Overweight and I Hate It" portrays the challenges encountered by a young man who is suffering because of his weight problem. This scenario may be used as a therapeutic tool to explore relationship difficulties and emotional issues involving nonacceptance of self and perceived or real rejection by others. Healthy life habits to replace harmful binge-eating could be discussed with clients in similar situations.

Additional Resources

Lock, J. (Ed.). (2011). *The Oxford handbook of child and adolescent eating disorders: Developmental perspectives.* New York: Oxford University Press.

Lock, J., & Le Grange, D. (2005). *Help your teenager beat an eating disorder.* New York: Guilford.

Ross, C. (2009). *The binge eating and compulsive overeating workbook: An integrated approach to overcoming disordered eating.* Oakland, CA: New Harbinger Publications, Inc.

Walsh, B. T., & Cameron, V. L. (2005). *If your adolescent has an eating disorder.* New York: Oxford University Press.

Healthy

I am really trying to improve myself. I am trying to be healthy. My family has trouble maintaining a healthy weight, so I am trying to be proactive. I don't want to be too thin or too overweight. I have been reading about foods that are good for me, like blueberries, fruit, and fish. I have even started eating more fruit and vegetables, and less fast food. Don't get me wrong, I still like my burgers and fries, but I am only having them once in awhile. I mean, I can't give up everything, right?

I've started to exercise too. I actually really like it. Sometimes I walk a mile or jog after school. What I really like is bike riding. When I'm doing something I like, I've found that I do it longer because I actually start having fun! Who knew that exercising could be so much fun? My friends Jordyn and Alex work out with me sometimes, which makes it even more fun than exercising alone. We listen to music or talk while we shoot baskets or jog at the recreation center. Then we will usually grab a healthy smoothie afterward. Who knew that being healthy could be so much fun? I usually feel in a great mood after the workout too!

Instructions: Tell, write, or draw the answers to the following questions.

Healthy Questions: Level 1

1. How is the person in this story feeling?
2. Is it healthy for this person to eat the way that he or she does?
3. Why is this person concerned about him or herself?
4. What are some other ways this person could be healthier?
5. What are some ways this person copes with stress?
6. What are some good things about this person?
7. How would you finish this story?

Healthy Questions: Level 2

1. Do you know anyone who is trying to be healthier?
2. What are his or her eating habits like?
3. What are his or her exercise habits like?
4. What does this person do to try to be healthier?
5. What are some good things about this person?
6. How would you finish his or her story?
7. How would you change his or her story if you could?

Healthy Questions: Level 3

1. Do you think you are healthy?
2. What are your eating habits like?
3. What could you do to make healthier choices?
4. What are your exercise habits like?

5. What are some ways you could cope with stress?
6. What are some good things about you?
7. How would you finish your story?
8. How would you change your story if you could?

My Story: Level 4

Instructions: Tell, write, or draw your own story.

I Think I'm Fat

I look in the mirror and I think I'm so fat. I can't stand it. Everyone tells me that I am not, but I know that I really am. I keep trying to lose more weight because I know I need to. I am one hundred pounds now but want to get down to ninety-five—then maybe I will finally look good.

My parents tell me that I am not eating enough, but I know that I am. They just don't understand. My friends are starting to really pester me too. My best friend even tried to force me to eat an ice cream cone! Can you believe that? I feel like everyone is against me. They got really mad at me the other day when I passed out—but how else am I going to lose this weight.

Maybe if I exercise even more, I'll reach my goal of ninety-five pounds. Then I would probably be happy and not feel and look so disgusting. I already get up before school to work-out. I run for three miles every morning and I make sure I skip breakfast. For lunch I eat an apple, which I think is healthy. My parents get furious with me when I eat only vegetables for dinner. They definitely just do not get me. They think I need to get professional help, and they say they care about me, but I think they are wrong.

Instructions: Tell, write, or draw the answers to the following questions.

I Think I'm Fat Questions: Level 1

1. How is the person in this story feeling?
2. Is it okay for this person to want to lose more weight?
3. Why are this person's friends and family concerned about him or her?
4. What are some ways this person could be healthy?
5. How would you finish this story?

I Think I'm Fat Questions: Level 2

1. Do you know anyone who has ever felt like he or she was overweight when he or she really was not overweight?
2. What did this person do to try to be thin?
3. Was this person making healthy choices?
4. What could this person do to try to be healthy?
5. How would you finish his or her story?
6. How would you change his or her story if you could?

I Think I'm Fat Questions: Level 3

1. Have you ever felt like you were overweight?
2. What did you do to try to lose weight?
3. Were you making healthy choices?
4. What are some healthy choices you could make?
5. How would you finish your story?
6. How would you change your story if you could?

My Story: Level 4

Instructions: Tell, write, or draw your own story.

I'm Overweight and I Hate It

Everyone tells me that I need to lose weight, even my friends and my parents. I know they are probably right, but I just can't seem to lose the weight. I just really love to eat! Food is my friend. I like a ton of junk food too. I love eating donuts, ice cream, and candy bars—sweets are my favorites. I really crave those all of the time. I like potato chips and tortilla chips too, but who doesn't? I find hot dogs and pepperoni pizza to be delicious too.

Sometimes I get depressed when something bad happens at school, like when I ask a girl out and she says no. This just happened yesterday. I approached Madison because she's so pretty and nice and asked her to go with me to the football game on Friday night. Of course she said no because she had other plans. After all, what did I really think she would say? Who wants to go out with a fat guy? She's probably dating some good-looking football player who is all muscular. Why would she possibly want me?

So after she told me that she wouldn't go out with me, I went home that night and just felt so horrible. I sat on the couch and watched a movie and ate—and ate and ate and ate. I ordered a pizza and ate the whole thing myself, and then I had a half-gallon of cookie dough ice cream, a bag of potato chips, two chocolate bars, and a two-liter bottle of pop. I felt kind of sickish afterward, but for a little while all of the food made me feel better—kind of like it didn't matter that Madison wouldn't date me . . .

The next day though, I looked in the mirror and felt horrible. I knew how much I ate last night and how bad it is for me, especially since I have type 2 diabetes. I wish I could stop eating, but it kind of makes me feel better, but then it makes me feel worse. I just weigh so much already, and it is like I just cannot stop. I don't know what I am going to do about my weight problem, and I definitely don't know how I'm ever going to get a girl to like me.

Instructions: Tell, write, or draw the answers to the following questions.

I'm Overweight and I Hate It Questions: Level 1

1. How is the person in this story feeling?
2. Is it okay for this person to eat the way that he does?
3. Why are this person's friends and family concerned about him?
4. What are some ways this person could be healthy?
5. What are some other ways this person could cope with stress besides eating?
6. What are some good things about this person?
7. How would you finish this story?

I'm Overweight and I Hate It Questions: Level 2

1. Do you know anyone who is overweight?
2. What are his or her eating habits like?
3. Is this person making healthy choices?
4. What does this person do to try to be healthier?
5. What are some good things about this person?

6. How would you finish his or her story?
7. How would you change his or her story if you could?

I'm Overweight and I Hate It Questions: Level 3

1. Do you think you are overweight?
2. What are your eating habits like?
3. What could you do to make healthier choices?
4. What are some ways you could cope with stress besides eating?
5. What are some good things about you?
6. How would you finish your story?
7. How would you change your story if you could?

My Story: Level 4

Instructions: Tell, write, or draw your own story.

12

Emotions

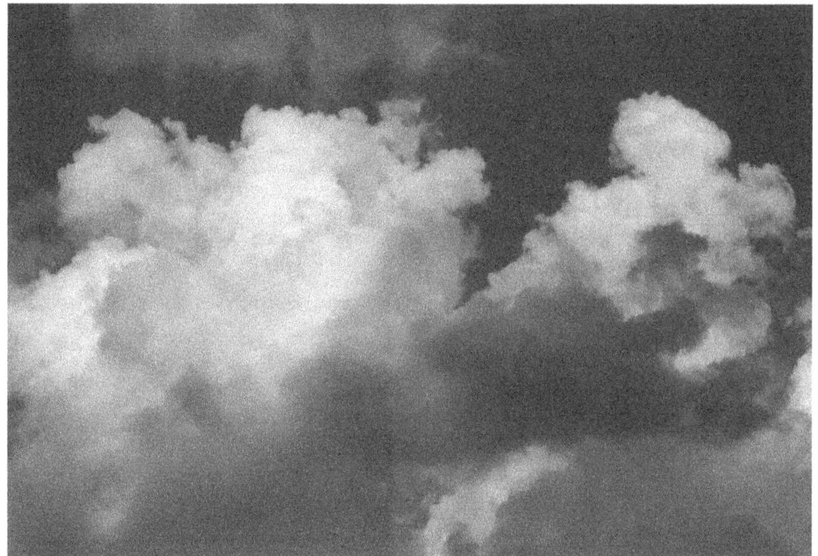

Key Practice Issues and Story Selection

Feelings of sadness, anger, and stress may contribute to teenagers' and young adults' feeling overwhelmed by life's challenges. All of these issues may play a part in the lowering of an individual's self-concept as well. Adolescents and young adults may need extra attention and support when traversing the unfamiliar territory of turbulent life choices and relationship hurdles. Many transitional life events may trigger periods of emotionality and temporary feelings of depression and anxiety. Others may face more long-term episodes of depression and anxiety that must be considered significant and addressed appropriately according to a given practitioner's style and methodology. Some of these events include but are not limited to:

- Dealing with the death of a friend, boyfriend or girlfriend, or family member
- Coping with the serious illness of a loved one or of oneself
- Transitioning from one school setting to another
- Facing academic, personal or professional challenges
- Dealing with relationship changes
- Entering into the world of work
- Being victimized as a result of sexual assault or abuse
- Experiencing parental divorce or separation

When faced with stressful or challenging life circumstances, individuals sometimes tend to maladaptively handle these events through either internalization or externalization. When internalizing, emotions may be kept tightly inside, which can contribute to feelings of anxiety, depression, and eating disorders. This tends to occur more often among adolescent females. When externalizing, individuals may act-out by driving too fast, punching walls, or behaving in an aggressive manner. Adolescent males are more likely to externalize their problems. However, remain cognizant that both females and males may internalize or externalize their emotional states and behaviors (Levine & Munsch, 2011; Newman & Newman, 2006).

Tips for practitioners assisting teenagers and young adults who experience difficulty in coping with feelings include:

- Teach individuals positive ways to manage or cope with their emotions by using techniques such as:
  - Journaling
  - Meditating
  - Exercising to relieve stress, anxiety, and depression
  - Sharing emotions with trusted friends, family, and therapists
  - Developing problem-solving skills (Carrell, 2000).
- Discuss with individuals that emotions in and of themselves are not bad, but people must learn to effectively express their emotions in socially acceptable and constructive manners.

The story "I'm So Depressed" portrays a situation in which a person feels misunderstood and abandoned by both friends and family members. Extreme sadness and depressed mood are demonstrated by the character's negative thoughts, feelings, and actions. These include withdrawing from healthy, enjoyable activities with others and crying excessively. Functioning in daily life has been impaired, and the character now feels that it is difficult to prepare for the day. School performance is also diminished.

Cognitive distortions could be challenged with the help of a professional, and adjunct referrals or treatments, in addition to storytelling, could be made as needed if a client is severely depressed.

Deep emotions of extreme sadness are vividly expressed in the scenario "The Pain," which is applicable to a variety of situations in a person's life. It could be applied to a person's life who is dealing with depression, but it also is applicable to feelings people may have after experiencing traumatic or frightening events or grief resulting from the death of a loved one. In addition, it could actually also apply to physical pain that a person experiences when suffering from a variety of illnesses or injuries. Some illnesses or injuries that can cause severe pain include rheumatoid arthritis, lupus, multiple sclerosis, amputations, cancer, traumatic brain injuries, neuropathy and other nerve related conditions, and the like. Healthy ways to cope with emotional and physical pain may be examined with the help of friends, family, and helping professionals.

"Life's So Unfair!" is a vignette in which the character explores how he or she feels angry, unheard, and uncared for by friends, family, and others. The validity of the experiences that evoke these feelings will vary from person to person, based on individual circumstances. Such feelings may be very legitimate in cases where social injustice such as discrimination based on gender, race, or sexual orientation is occurring. However, cognitive distortions may be present in the minds of some individuals, and reality testing may be beneficial for some individuals with the help of a mental health professional.

"Life Sucks!" is a brief scenario in which a person, who feels like he or she does not matter to anyone, feels badly about himself or herself. People who are encountering difficult times in their lives may relate to such feelings. Practitioners may encourage cathartic expression of emotion, as well as attempt to boost a person's self-esteem. If needed, methods to control one's anger may also be modeled and taught. Fostering of problem-solving and coping skills would also be of benefit.

"Cookie Storm" explores the feelings of a confused and overwhelmed teenager or young adult using the simile of his or her life being like a cookie storm smoothie. This fun analogy provides a nonthreatening way to discuss complicated emotions common during adolescence. Feelings of being "not normal" may be normalized through discussions explaining that others feel that way too.

Additional Resources

Berlinger, N. T. (2006). *Rescuing your teenager from depression.* New York: Harper Collins.

Evans, D. L., & Andrews, L. W. (2005). *If your adolescent has depression or bipolar disorder.* New York: Oxford University Press.

Foa, E. B., & Andrews, L. W. (2006). *If your adolescent has an anxiety disorder: An essential resource for parents.* New York: Oxford University Press.

Grant, J. E., & Potenza, M. N. (2009). *Young adult mental health.* New York: Oxford University Press.

I'm So Depressed

I am so depressed and I feel like no one understands me or what I am going through. I just come home from school and go to my room and lie in bed and cry. I don't know what is wrong with me. I feel like nobody likes me, and all of my old friends have abandoned me. They won't even hang out with me anymore or text me because I don't want to go anywhere or do anything with them right now. I feel like I've lost all of my friends.

I feel like the whole world is against me. My parents tell me to go outside and go for a walk, but I don't even have the energy to do that. I can barely run a brush through my hair in the morning, let alone take a shower. I really want to start feeling better, but I doubt that will ever happen. I just feel so hopeless. Now my grades are starting to drop too, and I used to be a really good student. This just makes me feel worse, like I'm a loser. I don't know what I am going to do.

Instructions: Tell, write, or draw the answers to the following questions.

I'm So Depressed Questions: Level 1

1. How is this person feeling?
2. Why does this person feel this way?
3. What could this person do to feel better?
4. How could this person reconnect with his or her friends?
5. How would you finish this story?

I'm So Depressed Questions: Level 2

1. Do you know anyone who has ever felt very sad or depressed?
2. Can you tell me what it is like for him or her to feel this way?
3. What does he or she do when he or she feels this way?
4. How does this person cope or how could this person cope with feeling so sad or depressed?
5. What is his or her story?
6. How would you change his or her story if you could?

I'm So Depressed Questions: Level 3

1. Have you ever felt very sad or depressed?
2. Can you tell me what it is like for you when you feel so badly?
3. How do you cope or how could you cope with feeling so sad or depressed?
4. How could you reconnect with your friends?
5. What is your story?
6. How would you change your story if you could?

My Story: Level 4

Instructions: Tell, write, or draw your own story.

The Pain

It hurts so badly and the pain's so fresh. I just rock myself to sleep at night and cry more and more to try to get all of the pain out of me. But the pain never seems to end. It's like an old friend that just keeps visiting and will never go away, even when you ask him to leave. It's like an old familiar soft, black cardigan that wraps around you when you are cold, and soothes you just enough to take away your chill. The pain just lingers and floats around in the space in my mind and infiltrates my heart. The pain keeps me company.

But the pain never really leaves. It is always there in the back of my mind, kind of haunting me, taunting me, and filling my spirit with sadness. I succumb to its greatness as it humbles me. Maybe someday someone will cast a magic spell on me to make it all disappear, and then I can go back in time and start my life all over again, one magical day at a time.

Instructions: Tell, write, or draw the answers to the following questions.

The Pain Questions: Level 1

1. How is this person feeling?
2. Why does this person feel this way?
3. What could this person do to feel better?
4. How could this person cope with the mental or physical pain he or she is experiencing?
5. How would you finish this story?

The Pain Questions: Level 2

1. Do you know anyone who has ever felt very much mental or physical pain?
2. Can you tell me what it is like for him or her to feel this way?
3. What does he or she do when he or she feels this way?
4. How does this person cope or how could this person cope with feeling so much pain?
5. What is his or her story?
6. How would you change his or her story if you could?

The Pain Questions: Level 3

1. Have you ever felt very much mental or physical pain?
2. Can you tell me what it is like for you when you feel so much pain?
3. How do you cope or how could you cope with feeling so much pain?
4. What are some good things about your body and mind?
5. What is your story?
6. How would you change your story if you could?

My Story: Level 4

Instructions: Tell, write, or draw your own story.

Life's So Unfair!

I'm so angry at everybody! Life is so unfair. I feel like everyone is always telling me what to do, but no one ever really wants to listen to what I have to say. They all say that they want to listen, but no one really ever does listen. They may hear my words, but they don't really hear what I am saying, nor do they care.

They all just tell me what to do without ever really asking what I really want in my own life. Why don't they care about what I want? I am a person too! They shouldn't ignore me—I have rights too! I feel like everyone is against me—my parents, my teachers, just everyone—I feel like telling them this is my life, and I will do whatever I want!

Instructions: Tell, write, or draw the answers to the following questions.

Life's So Unfair Questions: Level 1

1. Why is this person so angry?
2. What else is this person feeling?
3. What could this person do to feel better?
4. What does this person want out of his or her life?
5. How would you finish this story?

Life's So Unfair Questions: Level 2

1. Do you know anyone who has ever felt like the character in this story?
2. Can you tell me what it is like for him or her to feel this way?
3. What does he or she do when he or she feels this way?
4. How does this person deal with or how could this person deal with his or her feelings?
5. What is his or her story?
6. How would you change his or her story if you could?

Life's So Unfair Questions: Level 3

1. Have you ever felt like the character in the story?
2. Can you tell me what it is like for you when you feel angry, unheard, or ignored?
3. How does this make you feel?
4. What could you do to try to get people to hear what you are really saying?
5. What is your story?
6. How would you change your story if you could?

My Story: Level 4

Instructions: Tell, write, or draw your own story.

Life Sucks!

My life sucks! I feel like I hate everyone and I feel like I am such a loser. No one understands what I am going through, how could they? I have so much crap going on in my life right now that I wish everyone and everything would just go away. I wish I could become invisible, because that is how I feel. I might as well be invisible. No one pays attention to what I want anyway.

Maybe this is all just a bad dream because that is what my freaking life feels like . . .

Instructions: Tell, write, or draw the answers to the following questions.

Life Sucks Questions: Level 1

1. What is this person feeling?
2. What might this person have going on in his or her life right now?
3. What could this person do to feel less invisible and more seen?
4. What does this person want out of his or her life?
5. How would you finish this story?

Life Sucks Questions: Level 2

1. Do you know anyone who has ever felt like the character in this story?
2. Can you tell me what it is like for him or her to feel this way?
3. What does he or she do to cope when he or she feels this way?
4. How does this person deal with or how could this person deal with his or her feelings?
5. What is his or her story?
6. How would you change his or her story if you could?

Life Sucks Questions: Level 3

1. Have you ever felt like the character in the story?
2. Can you tell me what it is like for you when you feel invisible?
3. Can you tell me what it is like for you when you feel like a loser?
4. What could you do to try to get people to actually see the real you?
5. What is your story?
6. How would you change your story if you could?

My Story: Level 4

Instructions: Tell, write, or draw your own story.

Cookie Storm

I just can't handle my life! I feel like the walls of life are crumbling down around me like cookies crumbling in a blender. I don't know where I'm going in this cookie storm, nor do I know how I got here. I just know that I want the storm to end because I've got bits of chocolate chips stuck in my eyes and frosting in my hair. My life is such a mess—just like a big ice cream smoothie tornado that is ready to blow down the entire town!

Why can't I just be normal?

Instructions: Tell, write, or draw the answers to the following questions.

Cookie Storm Questions: Level 1

1. What is this person feeling?
2. What might this person have going on in his or her life right now?
3. What could this person do to feel more in control of his or her life?
4. What does this person want out of his or her life?
5. How would you finish this story?

Cookie Storm Questions: Level 2

1. Do you know anyone who has ever felt like the character in this story?
2. Can you tell me what it is like for him or her to feel this way?
3. What does he or she do to cope when he or she feels this way?
4. How does this person deal with or how could this person deal with his or her feelings?
5. What is his or her story?
6. How would you change his or her story if you could?

Cookie Storm Questions: Level 3

1. Have you ever felt like your life was out of control?
2. Can you tell me what it is like for you when you feel like your life is out of control?
3. What positive steps could you take to make your life better?
4. What are five good qualities that you have?
5. What is your story?
6. How would you change your story if you could?

My Story: Level 4

Instructions: Tell, write, or draw your own story.

13

Dating Violence

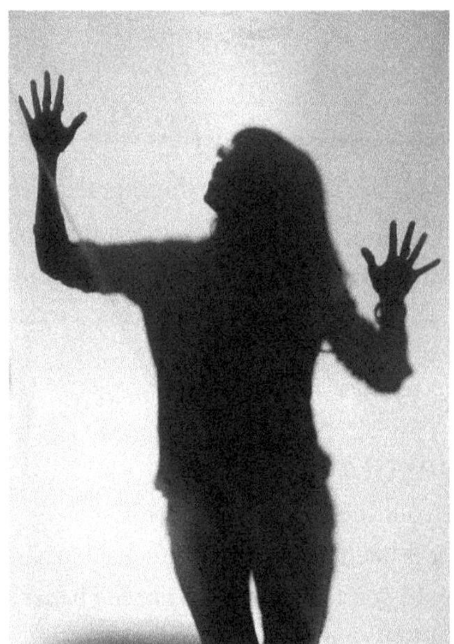

Key Practice Issues and Story Selection

Dating violence is something that many young adult females and adolescents will experience in their attempts to form intimate relationships. Young adult men and teenagers may experience it as well, in either heterosexual relationships or same-sex relationships. In any case, dating violence can be damaging to an individual's self-esteem at a minimum. It also may be dangerous, resulting in serious injury or death for the victims of dating violence.

According to Hickman and colleagues (2004), violence in dating relationships may take many forms, including:

- Verbal and emotional abuse (e.g. insults and derogatory name calling)
- Physical assault (e.g. hitting, slapping, or aggressively grabbing)
- Sexual assault (e.g. forcing someone to participate in unwanted sexual activity)
- Threatening to kill or actually murdering one's partner
- Killing the pets of a girlfriend or boyfriend
- Intimidating behavior (e.g. threatening romantic partners' loved ones)
- Stalking behavior (e.g. following a boyfriend or girlfriend in an automobile) (Hickman, Jaycox, & Aronoff, 2004)

Signs that a teen or young adult may be in an abusive relationship include but are not limited to:

- Controlling behavior on the part of the abusive partner (e.g. not letting the person engage in typical family or friendship activities)
- Extreme feelings of jealousy on the part of the violent partner (e.g. not letting the other person talk to other boys or girls)
- Submissive behavior on the part of the nonabusing partner
- Behavioral change on the part of the nonabusive partner

Many long-term relationships which exhibit serious issues involving one partner battering the other began as dating relationships. For this reason, practitioners must be aware of and remain vigilant to identify the signs of dating violence in adolescent and young adult relationships. General tips for practitioners include:

- Teaching nonviolent conflict resolution skills
- Teaching nonacceptance and rejection of violence in intimate relationships
- Identifying and reducing controlling and jealous behaviors (Ashford & LeCroy, 2010)

The story "I Love Him So Much" discusses common aspects and signs of relationships in which dating violence is occurring. It demonstrates how a person can be manipulated by controlling, possessive behavior. Also, verbal abuse involving derogatory name calling as well as physical abuse in the form of slapping and grabbing are shown. This story would be a valuable resource in practice with individuals who are current or past victims of dating violence, or when it is suspected that dating violence is happening. It may also be utilized preventively, to teach adolescents and young adults how to avoid being victims or perpetrators of intimate violence.

The next vignette, "The Texts," accurately portrays the distress and fear felt by a young woman whose ex-boyfriend is harassing her via texts. He simply will not leave her alone, even though she is ready to move on in her life without him. He also is threatening her and following her. This story could be used in the therapeutic setting to discuss safety planning for those who have left abusive relationships and to explore aspects of healthy versus unhealthy relationships and break-ups.

In "She Deserves It..." a young man expresses his feelings of extreme anger when his girlfriend breaks up with him. He also believes that she was unfaithful to him, and he is plotting revenge. This story could open the door for discussions with both young men and women in order to promote positive relationships skills, and healthy ways to cope after a relationship ends.

Additional Resources

Allen, M. (2012). *Narrative therapy for women experiencing domestic violence: Supporting women's transitions from abuse to safety.* London, UK: Jessica Kingsley.

Evans, P. (2010). *The verbally abusive relationship: How to recognize it and how to respond.* Avon, MA: Adams Media.

Nabors, E. L. (2010). Drug use and intimate partner violence among college students: An in-depth exploration. *Journal of Interpersonal Violence*, 25(6), 1043–1063. doi: 10.1177/0886260509340543

Nabors, E. L., & Jasinski, J. L. (2009). Intimate partner violence perpetration among college students: The role of gender role and gendered violence attitudes. *Feminist Criminology*, 4(1), 57–82. doi: 10.1177/1557085108325235

I Love Him So Much

I always thought that love was supposed to be such a great thing, but I just don't understand it at all. I think I love Ryan, and I know he says he loves me—and I think that he really does. But Ryan sure has a funny way of showing his love for me . . .

When we first started going out together, everything was great. He would text me sometimes and we would meet after school and hang out together. Sometimes we would go to the mall or go grab something to eat. He would take cool pictures of us and post them to his site, so all of our friends knew we were a couple. He even bought me roses on Valentine's Day to express his love for me. He was so sweet and made me feel really special.

After awhile though, he started getting really jealous when I talked to other boys in school and started giving us dirty looks. One day after school I was talking to Jacob in the hall, and he came up to me and called me a "slut." I couldn't believe it. I had no idea why he was acting that way, since he knew that I was friends with Jacob. He told me later that he was just so jealous because he loves me so much that he could not stand to see another guy talking to me. So now he doesn't even want me to talk to any of my friends who are guys.

Then, Alisha asked me to go to the football game with her on Friday night, and I said yes. So when I told Ryan I was going with Alisha to the game on Friday, he got really angry and started screaming at me. He said that I shouldn't be going out with my friends anymore, and that I should just be hanging out with him. He was so mad that I told him I would cancel my plans with Alisha on Friday, and go to the game with him. After all, I do love him and I don't want to lose him.

When we were walking around at the game, all kinds of trouble started when we saw my friend Austin. All that Austin did was say "hi" to me, so I said "hi" back to him and I smiled a friendly smile and so did Austin. We really are just friends. But after we walked away from Austin and his friends, Ryan grabbed me by my arm and pulled me into a corner and told me to never talk to Austin again. Then he slapped me across the face and I started to cry. I could hardly believe what was happening.

The next day he texted me and said how sorry he was. He said he loves me so much that he just goes crazy when he's around me. He promised that he'll never smack me again. I believe him—I have to, because I love him, and I forgive him. I really do love Ryan, but this relationship is really stressing me out!

Instructions: Tell, write, or draw the answers to the following questions.

I Love Him So Much Questions: Level 1

1. How is the girl in this story feeling?
2. Is it okay for Ryan to treat her the way he does?
3. Is it okay for the girl in this story to go out with her friends?
4. What are some characteristics of a healthy relationship?
5. How would you finish this story?

I Love Him So Much Questions: Level 2

1. Do you know anyone who has ever been in a very jealous or violent relationship?
2. How did this person feel about being in his or her relationship?
3. Did this person decide to stay in the relationship?
4. How would you finish his or her story?
5. How would you change his or her story if you could?

I Love Him So Much Questions: Level 3

1. Have you ever been in a very jealous or violent relationship?
2. Can you tell me what it was like for you being in a jealous or violent relationship?
3. Did you decide to stay in the relationship?
4. What are some of the positive and negative things about your current relationship?
5. What are some of your own strengths, not related to the relationship?
6. How would you finish your story?
7. How would you change your story if you could?

My Story: Level 4

Instructions: Tell, write, or draw your own story.

The Texts

He's texted me thirty times today—again. It's like he just won't quit. He knows I don't want to go out with him anymore, but he will not take no for an answer. He just will not leave me alone. He is really getting to me. He's not acting right, and he is starting to scare me. He's saying that he will hurt himself if I don't go back with him. What if he really did hurt himself? Then, in the very next text he will threaten me. He'll text things like "You'll be sorry if you don't get back with me," or "Don't ever let me catch you going out with another guy. You know what I'll do." What if he means it?

I would like to move on with my life, but he just won't leave me alone. I'm afraid of him. The other night he followed me when I drove to work. I could clearly see that it was him behind me in his red car. I don't know who to talk to about this. I don't know what to do.

Instructions: Tell, write, or draw the answers to the following questions.

The Texts Questions: Level 1

1. How is the girl in this story feeling?
2. Is it okay for her ex-boyfriend to treat her the way he does?
3. Is it okay for the girl in this story to move on with her life?
4. What are some characteristics of a healthy relationship?
5. How would you finish this story?

The Texts Questions: Level 2

1. Do you know anyone who has ever been in a very jealous or violent relationship?
2. How did this person feel about being in his or her relationship?
3. Did this person decide to stay in the relationship or to leave?
4. How would you finish his or her story?
5. How would you change his or her story if you could?

The Texts Questions: Level 3

1. Have you ever been in a very jealous or violent relationship?
2. Can you tell me what it was like for you being in a jealous or violent relationship?
3. Did you decide to stay in the relationship or did you leave?
4. What are some of the positive and negative things about your current relationship?
5. What are some of your own strengths, not related to the relationship?
6. How would you finish your story?
7. How would you change your story if you could?

My Story: Level 4

Instructions: Tell, write, or draw your own story.

She Deserves It...

She's such a bitch. She deserves what she gets for breaking up with me. I mean really, how could she do that to me? I'm so humiliated. She has no right to break up with me. I'm her boyfriend, not that other jerk.

I heard she even cheated on me. I'm going to get even with her. And I spent all of that money on her too. I even bought her a ring—I am so angry. When she goes out with him tonight I know what I am going to do . . .

Instructions: Tell, write, or draw the answers to the following questions.

She Deserves It Questions: Level 1

1. How is the boy in this story feeling?
2. Why is he so upset?
3. What do you think the boy in this story is thinking of doing? What will happen to him if he does this?
4. What are some characteristics of a healthy relationship?
5. How would you finish this story?

She Deserves It Questions: Level 2

1. Do you know anyone who has ever felt very angry that a girlfriend or boyfriend broke up with him or her?
2. How did this person handle the break-up?
3. How do you think he or she should have handled the break-up?
4. How would you finish his or her story?
5. How would you change his or her story if you could?

She Deserves It Questions: Level 3

1. Have you ever been very angry after your girlfriend or boyfriend broke up with you?
2. How did you handle the break-up?
3. How do you think you should have handled the break-up?
4. What are some of your own strengths, not related to a relationship?
5. How would you finish your story?
6. How would you change your story if you could?

My Story: Level 4

Instructions: Tell, write, or draw your own story.

14

Substance Abuse

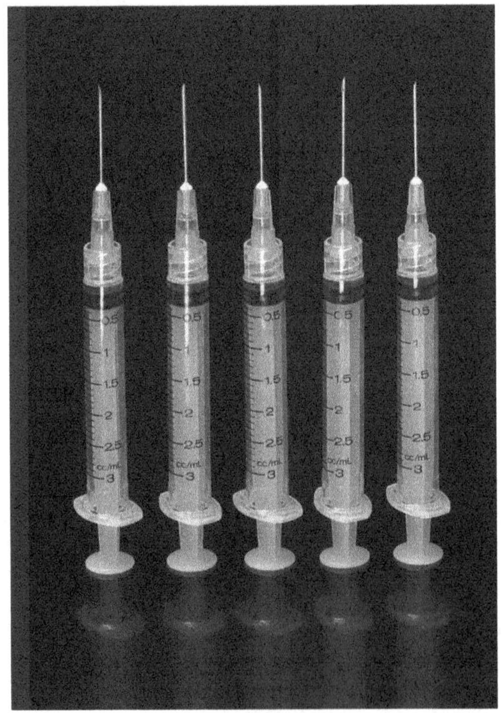

Key Practice Issues and Story Selection

Many teens and young adults will experiment with using drugs and alcohol as part of their developmental experience. Others, who may be predisposed genetically and because of life stressors or environmental circumstances, will rely on drug or alcohol use as a mainstay in their everyday lives. Some will become addicted to substances, which in turn will impact their current and future relationships, academic performance, career aspirations, and other important areas of life functioning.

Adolescence and young adulthood are high-risk periods for abuse of alcohol and drugs. Many will begin to drink alcohol in their early teens, perhaps as a combined result of the following contributing factors: peer pressure, imitation of parental drinking, easy access to alcohol, lack of supervision, and negative life events affecting adolescents' emotional states. Alcohol usage tends to increase during the teenage years and generally continues to increase as individuals enter young adulthood (Brown, et al., 2008).

Issues relevant to gender merit consideration when examining alcohol use among young adults. One longitudinal study of 166 adolescents who were tracked into young adulthood found that men were more likely to experience problematic drinking than were women. In addition, young men were found to be more likely to drink in dangerous situations, to drink excessively, and to become violent while drinking (Chartier, Hesselbrock, & Hesselbrock, 2011). Thus, when working with young men, potential implications of alcohol use should be considered and discussed, such as the potential to harm self and others, possible altercations with the police, and the risk of incarceration.

In the aforementioned study, notable differences regarding drinking habits were mentioned between those who were African American and those who were white. African Americans were more likely to begin having alcohol related problems at a later age than whites. These problems included arguing and physically fighting while intoxicated (for both African Americans and whites). In this particular study, overall, white men had the highest risk of developing serious problems stemming from alcohol compared to African American men or women and white women (Chartier, Hesselbrock, & Hesselbrock, 2011).

Various factors place adolescents and young people at risk for susceptibility to alcohol and drug abuse. A dynamic interplay of the following factors may contribute to difficulties with consuming substances and potential addictive behaviors:

- Desire to numb oneself from painful experiences or environments such as poverty, joblessness, or lack of education
- Lack of parental concern or supervision
- Parental use or abuse of drugs or alcohol
- Inadequately developed coping skills
- School or relationship challenges
- Thrill-seeking behavior
- Pressure from peers to fit-in (Dishion, Kavanagh, Schneiger, Nelson, & Kaufman, 2002; McWhirter, McWhirter, McWhirter & McWhirter, 2007)
- Past or current traumatic events such as sexual assault or child abuse

In the vignette "Recovery," a young adult is confronted with the reality of a mother's addiction. The character is hopeful yet cautious regarding a parent's recovery, as fear exists that relapses may ensue, or that treatment may be unsuccessful. Strengths of the individual are also mentioned, such as remaining focused on school and healthy aspects of one's life. Family stressors, addiction, and coping mechanisms may be explored when using this story therapeutically.

"Rehab" is a narrative in which a person reveals thoughts, emotions, and perceptions about what it is like to experience addiction counseling. Exploration of obstacles and strengths may occur when sharing this story with those struggling to surmount substance abuse challenges. Family members of chemically dependent individuals may benefit from hearing the perspective of someone transforming his or her life through treatment.

The story "High" describes what it is like to be addicted to drugs. Those who are addicted to various substances may relate to or identify with the main character. Those who are family members or friends of individuals addicted to substances may gain greater insight into the behavior and thought processes of those who are addicted to drugs or alcohol. Insight into self may also be gained.

"The Baller" is a vignette that addresses issues, concerns, and very real dangers that arise when a young person is entangled in the frightening world of dealing drugs. Although the character in this story is a drug dealer, the human side of his or her character is conveyed, especially when he or she worries about how disappointed his or her grandma would feel if she found out about the drug dealing. Also, legal issues and implied risk of bodily harm or death are addressed. This story could be used with those who glorify drug dealers to examine the very real risks involved in such a dangerous and illegal activity.

Additional Resources

Diamond, J. (2002). *Narrative means to sober ends: Treating addiction and its aftermath.* New York: Guilford.

Epstein, E. E., & McCrady, B. S. (2009). *Overcoming alcohol use problems: A cognitive-behavioral treatment program.* New York: Oxford University Press.

Gossop, M. (2003). *Drug Addiction and its treatment.* New York: Oxford University Press.

van Wormer, K., & Davis, D. R. (2008). *Addiction treatment: A strengths perspective.* Belmont, CA: Thomson Brooks/Cole.

Recovery

My mom went to rehab and now she's in recovery. I'm very proud of her for quitting drinking. She used to really drink a lot and when she was drunk she would say such stupid things. She would embarrass me so badly in front of my friends. I felt so ashamed. It was extremely difficult for me and for all of my family to handle. She has asked us all to forgive her, and we are trying to, but it is really hard to because she has just hurt us so badly. She has been mean sometimes when she was drunk, and that is just impossible to forget. I do still love her though—I mean, she still is my mom. I just hope she can stay sober this time. I suppose we will wait and see what happens. If she can't stay sober, I will just have to stay focused on me, my friends, and school. Really, what else can I do?

Instructions: Tell, write, or draw the answers to the following questions.

Recovery Questions: Level 1

1. How is this person feeling?
2. What might this person have going on in his or her life right now?
3. Can you relate to how this person is feeling?
4. How can this person cope with a parent's addiction?
5. What does this person want out of his or her life?
6. How would you finish this story?

Recovery Questions: Level 2

1. Do you know anyone who has had a family member in recovery?
2. Can you tell me what it was like for his or her family when he or she was in recovery?
3. What does this person have going on in his or her life?
4. Did this person's family member ever stop using alcohol or drugs?
5. What is his or her story?
6. How would you change his or her story if you could?

Recovery Questions: Level 3

1. Has a family member of yours ever been in recovery?
2. Can you tell me what it was like for you when the family member was in recovery?
3. What did you or do you have going on in your life?
4. What positive steps could you take to cope with a family member's addiction?
5. What are five good qualities that you have?
6. Did your family member ever stop using alcohol or drugs?
7. What is your story?
8. How would you change your story if you could?

My Story: Level 4

Instructions: Tell, write, or draw your own story.

Rehab

I had to go rehab, and it was so intense. I suppose it was a good thing I went. I had been using every day and was getting into some pretty dangerous situations, but I felt like I just didn't care. It seemed like nothing really mattered to me. Everything I cared about before just seemed to be slipping away from my life. In rehab, we had group therapy twice a day and they made us talk about our feelings, all of the reasons we use, and how we could develop healthier coping mechanisms besides drinking and drugs. They taught us to be responsible for ourselves and for our actions. We had to make amends to those we had hurt. Some people forgave me, but some did not. That was really hard to know that I had hurt people so badly when I was drunk or high that they couldn't forgive me. But I am learning to cope and how to move on with life in a more positive way. I will learn from my mistakes, and I am starting to feel healthier mentally and physically already. I hadn't realized what a mess my life had become! Sometimes though, I still have bad cravings to drink or to use. I wish those cravings would go away. I hope I can stay clean and don't end up back in rehab. My family will be so mad at me if I relapse. I am making sure I am going to meetings every week and seeing my outpatient counselor often. I think maybe I can make it through this.

Instructions: Tell, write, or draw the answers to the following questions.

Rehab Questions: Level 1

1. How is this person feeling?
2. What might this person have going on in his or her life right now?
3. Can you relate to how this person is feeling?
4. Do you think this person might have a problem with addiction or drug use?
5. What does this person want out of his or her life?
6. How would you finish this story?

Rehab Questions: Level 2

1. Do you know anyone who has ever been to rehab?
2. Can you tell me what it was like for him or her to be in rehab?
3. What does this person have going on in his or her life?
4. Did this person ever stop using alcohol or drugs?
5. What is his or her story?
6. How would you change his or her story if you could?

Rehab Questions: Level 3

1. Have you ever gone to rehab?
2. Can you tell me what it was like for you in rehab?
3. What did you or do you have going on in your life?
4. What positive steps could you take to make your life better?

5. What are five good qualities that you have?
6. Did you ever stop using alcohol or drugs?
7. What is your story?
8. How would you change your story if you could?

My Story: Level 4

Instructions: Tell, write, or draw your own story.

High

Man, I just want to get high . . . I've got to find some pot. I just want to make it all disappear. All of the crap in my life just melts away when I am high, and all of the bad things just seem like an old forgotten bad dream. When I'm not high, I just want to get high. Do you know anybody I can buy from? If he doesn't have any pot, I'll take some pills or whatever he's got. If you don't know anybody, I'm just going to raid the medicine cabinet.

I just want to get high. I'm really jones'n.

Instructions: Tell, write, or draw the answers to the following questions.

High Questions: Level 1

1. How is this person feeling?
2. What might this person have going on in his or her life right now?
3. Can you relate to how this person is feeling?
4. Do you think this person might have a problem with addiction or drug use?
5. What does this person want out of his or her life?
6. How would you finish this story?

High Questions: Level 2

1. Do you know anyone who has ever felt like he or she needed to get high?
2. Can you tell me what it is like for him or her to feel this way?
3. What does this person have going on in his or her life?
4. Did this person ever stop using drugs?
5. What is his or her story?
6. How would you change his or her story if you could?

High Questions: Level 3

1. Have you ever felt like you needed to get high?
2. Can you tell me what it is like for you when you felt this way?
3. What did you or do you have going on in your life?
4. What positive steps could you take to make your life better?
5. What are five good qualities that you have?
6. Did you ever stop using drugs?
7. What is your story?
8. How would you change your story if you could?

My Story: Level 4

Instructions: Tell, write, or draw your own story.

The Baller

I can't believe I'm walking around with $5,000 in my pocket right now. If my grandma knew what I'm doing she would kill me. Well Grandma will never find out...I just have to make sure this gets delivered on time to Mr. Shade or we'll all go down for this as a bad deal. Trust me—none of us want that.

I'm more worried about Mr. Shade and his bangers than I am about the police. At least if the police catch me, I'll just end up in jail for a time. I know plenty of guys that are in. If Mr. Shade and his guys get cranked up, I think we all know what they'll do to us.

Instructions: Tell, write, or draw the answers to the following questions.

The Baller Questions: Level 1

1. What kind of activities is this person involved in?
2. What are some of the consequences or risks that this person is facing for drug dealing?
3. Can you relate to how this person is feeling?
4. Do you think this person might have a problem with addiction or drug use?
5. What does this person want out of his or her life?
6. How would you finish this story?

The Baller Questions: Level 2

1. Do you know anyone who has ever been involved in activities like dealing drugs?
2. What were some of the consequences or risks that this person faced for drug dealing?
3. What does this person have going on in his or her life?
4. Did this person have a problem with addiction or drug use?
5. Did this person ever get his or her life together? If so, how did this person improve his or her life?
6. What is his or her story?
7. How would you change his or her story if you could?

The Baller Questions: Level 3

1. Have you ever been involved in activities like dealing drugs?
2. What were some of the consequences or risks that you faced for drug dealing?
3. What did you have going on in your life?
4. Did you have a problem with addiction or drug use?
5. What positive steps did you or could you take to get your life together?
6. What is your story?
7. How would you change your story if you could?

My Story: Level 4

Instructions: Tell, write, or draw your own story.

15

Trauma

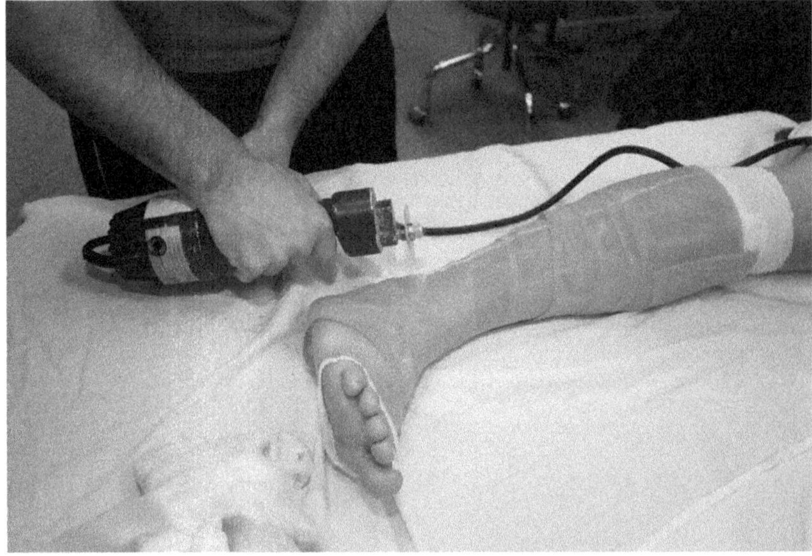

Key Practice Issues and Story Selection

Adolescence and young adulthood are periods in which many individuals will engage in high-risk behaviors that often will lead to negative, painful consequences. These traumatic consequences include such distressing events such as automobile and motorcycle accidents, shootings, and accidents or injuries from falls or stunts. In fact, for teenagers, some of the leading causes of brain injury include:

- Participation in sports
- Automobile accidents
- Engaging in dangerous behaviors, such as performing extreme stunts (Leone, 2011)

Among those between the ages of 10 and 24 in the United States, 71% of deaths occur because of four primary causes: vehicular crashes (31%), other unintentional injuries (14%), murder (15%), and suicide (11%) (Centers for Disease Control, NCHS, 2006). These same behaviors can contribute to serious injuries, disabilities, and post-traumatic stress disorder among adolescents and young adults. Post-traumatic stress disorder may occur when someone has been a direct recipient or witness to a particular traumatic event. It may also occur when someone has learned of a devastating event that has occurred to a valued loved one (Weis, 2008). Currently in the United States, "the most common traumatic events involving youth include exposure to violent crime, auto accidents, home fires and injuries, natural disasters, domestic violence, physical and sexual abuse, and serious physical illnesses" (Weis, 2008, p. 461). Internationally and within the United States, exposure to fighting, gunfire, explosions, and sexual assault, along with a general feeling of being unsafe from living in a war-torn area or from active combat, may cause people to experience significant stress and consequences as a result of witnessing or being a direct victim of violence. Many adolescents and young adults throughout the world encounter war or combat-related trauma on a regular basis.

Natural disasters such as earthquakes, hurricanes, tsunamis, floods, tornadoes, and fires also impact the survivors of these devastating events. Their needs and concerns may vary, depending on the level of devastation experienced by victims. Many may need immediate assistance for provision of basic needs such as food, clean water, clothing, and shelter at the time of the disaster itself. Medical care may also be required. These necessities are vital in this dire time of need, and may serve as a basis for rebuilding the foundation of transformed and displaced lives. Later, as victims are sometimes relocated to shelters, trailers, tents, or hotels, an additional adjustment period may be experienced, as well as possible mourning for loss of home, place, and material items. Clinicians may at times serve as an integral mental health member of a first responder team. In addition, many mental health practitioners will assist clients and families later in their recovery journey, as they muddle through their memories of the traumatic event and adjust to their current state of existence. Some individuals may experience long-term effects that result in the diagnosis of post-traumatic stress disorder.

People who experience post-traumatic stress may feel afraid, loss of control, helpless, and terror (Weis, 2008). This is likely to contribute to symptoms such as:

- Having flashbacks or nightmares involving a traumatic event such as a car accident or natural disaster
- Feeling agitated, irritable, or angry, especially when exposed to reminders of the event, such as a television show about tornadoes or earthquakes
- Feeling detached from loved ones
- Feeling easily startled

- Avoiding people and places associated with the traumatic event, such as not wanting to drive down a road where an accident occurred
- Feeling like there is no or little hope for the future (American Psychiatric Association, *DSM-IV-TR*, 2000)

Use of art therapy and storytelling techniques may be particularly helpful for adolescents who have experienced traumatic events, as they may avoid talking about the trauma. They may emotionally distance themselves from loved ones and may become isolated in attempts to shield themselves from the pain (Weis, 2008). Practitioners may gently encourage the release of emotions through the use of expressive arts and narrative.

In "The Storm," a young adult survives a terrible storm, such as a hurricane. This person recounts how living through this storm has affected him or her, as well as loved ones. In practice, it could be utilized to explore emotions surrounding the traumatic events of a natural disaster, as well as issues involving relocation and shelter living. Hope may be fostered by examining factors that enable people to overcome difficult situations, such as assisting in the provision of food, housing, and emotional support.

The scenario, "The Crash," describes a traumatic automobile accident involving a high rate of speed and drinking while driving. The character and others involved in the accident are injured and deeply affected by this preventable event. This story could be used preventatively with teens and young adults to discourage reckless behaviors such as drunk driving and speeding. It also could be used as a treatment tool to allow for expression of emotions surrounding similar tragedies.

In the story "The Tornado," a young person continues to suffer symptoms of post-traumatic stress long after a natural disaster has occurred. Those who have experienced a natural disaster may relate to this story. Expression of frightening memories and emotions should be encouraged, as well as exploring positive development of coping mechanisms to aid in handling this type of traumatic and devastating natural disaster.

Additional Resources

Cohen, J. A., Mannarino, A. P., & Deblinger, E. (2006). *Treating trauma and traumatic grief in children and adolescents.* New York: Guilford Press.

Heller, L., & Lapierre, A. (2012). *Healing developmental trauma: How early trauma affects self-regulation, self-image, and the capacity for relationship.* Berkeley, CA: North Atlantic Books.

Levers, L. L. (2012). *Trauma counseling: Theories and interventions.* New York: Springer.

Matthes-Loy, C. (2011). *Narrative therapy for posttraumatic stress disorder: Narrative change and symptom reduction.* Chicago, IL: UMI Dissertation Publishers.

The Storm

We knew the storm would be coming, but we had no idea it would be this bad. Debris and glass were flying everywhere and then came the flooding. We had the windows shuttered, and that helped some but it did nothing to prevent the flooding. It is just such a mess and some of our special things got ruined or lost. I can't even find the bracelet that Caden gave me because it was washed away in all of the water. My little sister misses her special teddy bear. She used to sleep with it every night. We even had to go onto the roof to be rescued, which was really scary because the floodwaters were flowing so fast. Now I don't know where we will stay—maybe in a shelter for awhile. How scary…I just want to go home, but there is no way we can go back home right now. The water is still too high and they say the area is contaminated, whatever that means.

I am just so glad we are all safe. I don't know what we will do now, but if I keep my head on straight I suppose I can handle this. It is very stressful, but some people are being really nice. After they rescued us, the organization that helped us gave us food and drinks. A counselor was there to talk to us too. Then they gave my little sister a new teddy bear, and their kindness made us all feel a little bit better.

Instructions: Tell, write, or draw the answers to the following questions.

The Storm Questions: Level 1

1. How is the person in the story feeling?
2. Why is he or she so upset?
3. How can this person cope with the aftereffects of the storm?
4. How would you finish this story?

The Storm Questions: Level 2

1. Do you know anyone who has ever experienced a storm or other natural disaster?
2. Can you tell me about what happened in his or her situation?
3. How did he or she cope with what happened to him or her?
4. What is his or her story?
5. How would you change his or her story if you could?

The Storm Questions: Level 3

1. Have you ever experienced a storm or other natural disaster?
2. Can you tell me about what happened and how you felt?
3. Who did you turn to for help regarding what happened?
4. What are your strengths that can help you to cope with your situation?
5. What is your story?
6. How would you change your story if you could?

My Story: Level 4

Instructions: Tell, write, or draw your own story.

The Crash

It was so scary last night. A bunch of us guys were out last night just messing around—about eight of us. We were in our cars and started racing and had been drinking some too. We were having really a lot of fun until it happened. We were speeding incredibly fast when Derek lost control. Then Derek wrecked into Mason's car. The crash was horrific—it was so loud, and people were crying, screaming, and moaning. There was blood everywhere, and hair and skin were stuck in the dashboard. They had to cut the car open to get Derek out. Most of us got pretty messed up. They told me I was lucky I didn't get killed. In fact, I'm posting this from the hospital right now.

As you can see, I have bandages all ever my head and my leg is broken. I need surgery tomorrow. This really sucks. I suppose I am the lucky one though. Derek has a head injury and is in a coma. They don't know if he will make it or not. I could hear his parents crying out in the hallway. How could we have been so stupid?

Instructions: Tell, write, or draw the answers to the following questions.

The Crash Questions: Level 1

1. How is the young man in the story feeling?
2. Why is he so upset?
3. How can this boy cope with what has happened to him and his friends?
4. How would you finish this story?

The Crash Questions: Level 2

1. Do you know anyone who has ever been in a very bad car accident?
2. Can you tell me about what happened in his or her situation?
3. How did he or she cope with what happened to him or her?
4. What did he or she learn from the accident?
5. What is his or her story?
6. How would you change his or her story if you could?

The Crash Questions: Level 3

1. Have you ever been in a very bad car accident?
2. Can you tell me about what happened and how you felt?
3. Who did you turn to for help regarding what happened?
4. What are your strengths that can help you to cope with your situation?
5. What is your story?
6. How would you change your story if you could?

My Story: Level 4

Instructions: Tell, write, or draw your own story.

The Tornado

Every time I hear the wind blow or hear a crack of thunder I just start to freak out. And if it starts to hail like it did the day of the storm, I just completely lose it. Sometimes I still can't believe that it ever really happened. I mean you see it on the news a lot around April or May, but you never really think it's going to happen to you and your family. When the storm came, it just ripped right through our town. So much was totally destroyed.

Now it is like I can't escape it. I get so nervous about the littlest of things. I wish I could make the whole experience just go away.

Instructions: Tell, write, or draw the answers to the following questions.

The Tornado Questions: Level 1

1. How is the person in the story feeling?
2. Why is he or she so upset?
3. How can this person cope with the aftereffects of the tornado?
4. How would you finish this story?

The Tornado Questions: Level 2

1. Do you know anyone who has ever experienced a tornado or other natural disaster?
2. Can you tell me about what happened in his or her situation?
3. How did he or she cope with what happened to him or her?
4. What is his or her story?
5. How would you change his or her story if you could?

The Tornado Questions: Level 3

1. Have you ever experienced a tornado or other natural disaster?
2. Can you tell me about what happened and how you felt?
3. Who did you turn to for help regarding what happened?
4. What are your strengths that can help you to cope with your situation?
5. What is your story?
6. How would you change your story if you could?

My Story: Level 4

Instructions: Tell, write, or draw your own story.

16

Military Issues and International Violence

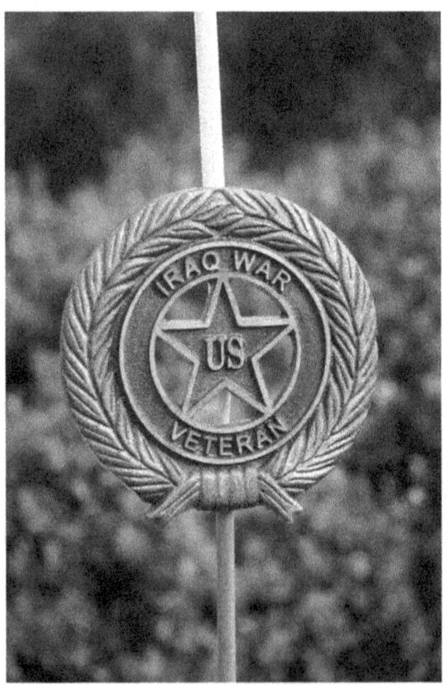

Key Practice Issues and Story Selection

Many teenagers and young adults have family members, friends, boyfriends or girlfriends, and spouses who actively serve or have served in the military. When a loved one or family member serves, the impact of service to one's country can impact all members of a family in unique ways. Experiencing feelings of ambivalence are not uncommon.

Although family members, relatives, and friends may feel proud of a person's sacrifice, honor, and bravery, they may simultaneously feel anger, disappointment, and sadness that the person is missing significant life events in the scope of their lives. They may also worry about the safe return of their loved one, and consider the possible losses from physical and mental disability or even death. Many young men and women have actively served and sacrificed for their country. Some may return with physical or mental challenges associated or directly caused from injuries endured while serving in the military.

When a loved one returns from deployment, additional relationship challenges may then be faced. After serving in war-time, a person may feel, act, and behave very differently than prior to deployment. He or she may experience symptoms of depression, anxiety, anger, and post-traumatic stress syndrome. Various physical and mental disabilities, including traumatic brain injury or amputations, may also be present. All of these mental and physical obstacles may impact current and future relationships with children, intimate partners, friends, and other family members. Many individuals and families could benefit from services provided by helping professionals (U. S. Department of Veteran Affairs, National Center for PTSD, 2009).

Everyone reacts in his or her own unique way to a loved one's deployment based on key factors such as relationship to the deployed person, age and developmental level of the person left behind, and co-occurring stressors. The following information about young adults and adolescents is summarized from an article provided by the United States Department of Veteran Affairs and its National Center for PTSD (2009). For young adults who may be married, the person left behind may feel:

- Overwhelmed
- Anxious
- Lonely
- Depressed
- Worried about financial and other responsibilities
- Fearful for the wellbeing of their loved one

For those in adolescence, it is not uncommon for young people to exhibit the following reactions to a parent's deployment:

- Feeling angry (e.g. punching the wall)
- Behaviorally acting out (e.g. driving the car too fast or using drugs)
- Becoming socially withdrawn and isolated (e.g. not wanting to leave one's room)
- Acting like he or she does not care about anything (e.g. making comments like, "It doesn't matter to me that Dad's gone")
- Losing interest in activities that were once enjoyed (e.g. making comments like, "I don't want to go running anymore")

In the story "Afghanistan," a young woman is worried and anxious regarding her boyfriend's deployment to Afghanistan. She is justifiably upset and concerned about the possibilities of him being seriously injured or killed in the line of duty. Comfort and support could be provided to those who relate to this difficult scenario, while ways of coping could be discussed in the context of the therapeutic setting.

"My Dad's Deployment" addresses the ambivalent feelings a teenager has regarding a parent serving in the military. While the character is proud of his or her father for sacrificing for his country, he or she also feels devastated that he will be missing very important parts of his or her life, such as not being available to help teach the character to drive a car. Those who identify with this story may benefit by realizing that they are not the only people to have mixed and confusing feelings about a parent's military deployment.

"Tour of Duty" examines the thoughts and feelings surrounding a person experiencing the aftereffects of military service. These include symptoms related to exposure to a traumatic event, such as hypervigilance and nightmares. It addresses the adjustment process and ensuing difficulties when returning to civilian life after deployment. Coping mechanisms could be taught and integrated into co-narrated stories related to successful adaptation and readjustment into society.

Additional Resources

Blaisure, K. R., Saathoff-Wells, T., Pereira, A., Wadsworth, S. M., & Dombro, A. L. (2012). *Serving military families in the 21st century.* New York: Routledge.

Cox, D., & Pawar, M. (2006). *International social work: Issues, strategies, and programs.* Thousand Oaks, CA: Sage.

Schauer, M., Neuner, F., & Elbert, T. (Eds.). (2005). *Narrative exposure therapy (NET): A short-term intervention for traumatic stress disorders after war, terror, or torture.* Cambridge, MA: Hogrefe.

Schauer, M., Neuner, F., & Elbert, T. (2011). *Narrative exposure therapy: A short-term treatment for traumatic stress disorders.* Cambridge, MA: Hogrefe.

Afghanistan

My boyfriend's in Afghanistan and I really, really, miss him badly. I can't wait until he comes home so we can get married. He's a great guy and I'm so proud of him. He is doing what he always has wanted to do; he's protecting our country from terrorism and is fighting for freedom. Sometimes I worry about him though, because he has seen some fighting...What if he comes back injured? Or worse yet, what if he doesn't come back at all?

I have thought about how horrible it would be to lose him. He just tells me to hang tight and wait for him. I know he'll be home soon . . .

Instructions: Tell, write, or draw the answers to the following questions.

Afghanistan Questions: Level 1

1. What is this young woman so concerned about?
2. What else is this person feeling?
3. What could this person do to cope with this difficult situation?
4. Who can she turn to for support?
5. How would you finish this story?

Afghanistan Questions: Level 2

1. Do you know anyone who has ever missed and worried about someone who was fighting in a war?
2. Can you tell me what it was like for him or her to feel this way?
3. What did the person do to help him or her to cope with this difficult situation?
4. Who did he or she turn to for support?
5. What is his or her story?
6. How would you change his or her story if you could?

Afghanistan Questions: Level 3

1. Have you ever missed and worried about someone who was fighting in a war?
2. Can you tell me what it was like for you to feel this way?
3. What did you do or what could you do to help you cope with this difficult situation?
4. Who did you or can you turn to for support?
5. What is your story?
6. How would you change your story if you could?

My Story: Level 4

Instructions: Tell, write, or draw your own story.

My Dad's Deployment

Well, Dad got the call today that his Air Force Reserve Unit is being deployed. All I could think about was "Why do we have to go through this all over again?" Don't get me wrong, I am extremely proud of my father and his service and sacrifice for our country. I just don't want him to go away again, and I don't want to have to worry about him and whether or not he will return safely.

Everything just seems harder when he is away—and I feel like he misses these big gaps in my life. Hopefully, I'll be getting my driver's license this year, but I guess he probably won't be here to teach me. I suppose Mom or Uncle Jake can help me. It's just not the same as Dad being here. I know I sound selfish, but I really don't want him to go.

Instructions: Tell, write, or draw the answers to the following questions.

My Dad's Deployment Questions: Level 1

1. What is this young person so concerned about?
2. What emotions is this person feeling?
3. What could this person do to cope with this difficult situation?
4. Who can he or she turn to for support?
5. How would you finish this story?

My Dad's Deployment Questions: Level 2

1. Do you know anyone who has ever missed and worried about someone who was deployed or fighting in a war?
2. Can you tell me what it is like for him or her to feel this way?
3. What did the person do to help him or her to cope with this difficult situation?
4. Who did he or she turn to for support?
5. What is his or her story?
6. How would you change his or her story if you could?

My Dad's Deployment Questions: Level 3

1. Have you ever missed and worried about someone who was deployed or fighting in a war?
2. Can you tell me what it is like for you to feel this way?
3. What did you do or what could you do to help you cope with this difficult situation?
4. Who did you or can you turn to for support?
5. What is your story?
6. How would you change your story if you could?

My Story: Level 4

Instructions: Tell, write, or draw your own story.

Tour of Duty

Things haven't been right since I got back from my last tour. I am tired all of the time and am jumpy. I haven't been able to sleep well because of those constant nightmares. It is the same horrible dream most nights. I always see the truck ahead of mine explode in our convoy and hear the screams of my friends as they become injured right before my eyes. Each night I have that dream I try to tell them to take a different route or to go left instead of right at that spot on that narrow, sandy road, but to no avail. My ears still ring from that awful explosion. I just know something bad is going to happen to me, as it usually does when I get that feeling. My family and friends are becoming worried about me, but I just can't seem to have a serious conversation with them as no one seems to appreciate all that I have done to make this world a safer place.

Instructions: Tell, write, or draw the answers to the following questions.

Tour of Duty Questions: Level 1

1. What happened to the person in this story?
2. What is this person feeling?
3. What could this person do to cope with this difficult situation?
4. Who can he or she turn to for support?
5. How would you finish this story?

Tour of Duty Questions: Level 2

1. Do you know anyone who has ever been in a war?
2. Can you tell me what it is like for him or her to actively serve in the military?
3. How did the person cope with his or her experiences?
4. Who did he or she turn to for support?
5. What is his or her story?
6. How would you change his or her story if you could?

Tour of Duty Questions: Level 3

1. Have you ever been in a war?
2. Can you tell me what it was like for you?
3. What did you do or what could you do to help you cope?
4. Who did you or can you turn to for support?
5. What is your story?
6. How would you change your story if you could?

My Story: Level 4

Instructions: Tell, write, or draw your own story.

17

Death

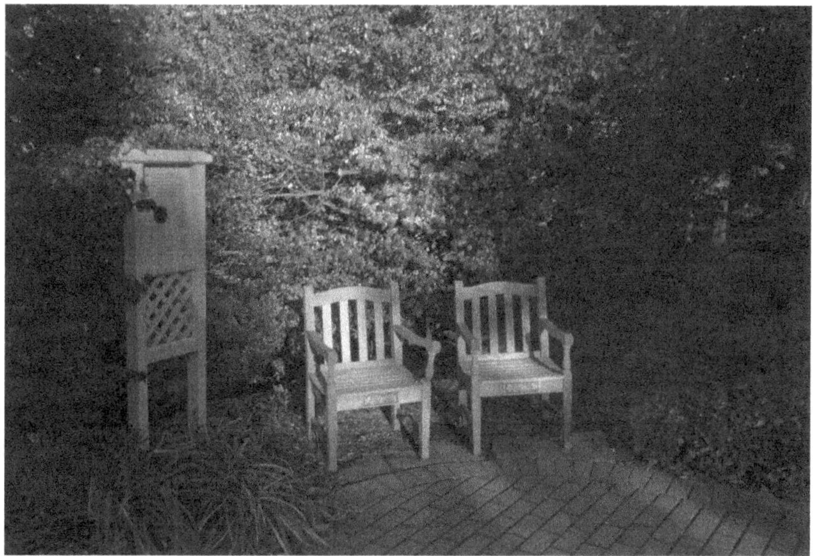

Key Practice Issues and Story Selection

Sadly, one hardship that many adolescents and young adults will encounter is the death of a loved one. The loss of friends and family members is difficult for anyone to endure, but it may be complicated by additional developmental crises, such as trying to solidify one's own identity or attempting to nurture an intimate relationship. If multiple losses occur in close proximity, this may contribute to even more difficulties in coping. For some individuals, this may lead to "bereavement overload and may cause the grieving process to shut down or to manifest itself in various somatic symptoms" (Worden, 2009, p. 210).

For example, if a teenager is already experiencing much confusion about who he or she really is, and is acting out toward his or her parent, and then the parent dies, this will undoubtedly further complicate the situation. This situation could then be further compounded if additional losses occur, such as the death of close friends in a traumatic car accident. Somatic symptoms such as headaches, pains, or frequent illness may also develop. These types of experiences may leave a teenager or young adult feeling emotionally devastated or emotionally numb—either of which may require additional support from a helping professional. Providing extra comfort in the midst of trauma while actively promoting healthy coping remains crucial.

In many instances for adolescents the expression of grief and the consequential experience of mourning are typical after the death of a loved one. Many individuals may not require professional help, whereas for others a similar loss serves as a catalyst igniting a negative, maladaptive reaction. In the latter circumstance, assistance from compassionate professionals could be of great benefit. Remain cognizant that bereavement is a highly individualized process (Blundell, 2001).

Everyone grieves differently depending on various factors, including temperament, personality, culture, religion, gender, developmental stage, and so forth. Some people may express themselves in a very emotional manner such as crying, sobbing, or talking; others may less openly explore their emotions. In general, adolescent boys act-out more and become destructive after the loss of a loved one. Teenage girls, however, are more apt to experience depression and isolation. Bereavement may exacerbate pre-existing challenges or issues such as loneliness, substance abuse, eating disorders, anxiety, and depression. In addition, unresolved issues from childhood may resurface and contribute to emotional vulnerability because of the death of a parent, friend, or relative. When treating adolescents, drawing may serve as a less threatening means of emotional release while revealing their innermost views and emotions (Blundell, 2001).

As unique human beings, everyone interprets and experiences death and the grieving process through his or her own lens of individualized feelings, thoughts, and perceptions. Individual experiences of grief will vary and are influenced by the following:

- Situational circumstances surrounding the death (e.g. gunshot wound, prolonged cancer, car accident, sudden heart attack)
- Age of the deceased (e.g. was the death of an older person or of a child or teenager)
- Developmental stage of the bereaved (e. g. a teenager is likely to interpret death in a different manner and will be affected differently than an older adult)
- Relationship to the deceased (e.g. when feelings of deep attachment and love exist, a person is likely to experience intense feelings of sadness and loss; however, grief may be difficult and complicated when relationships are conflicted or adversarial)

A classic theory regarding death and dying was developed by Elisabeth Kübler-Ross in 1969 after studying the experiences of those living with terminal illnesses. She later formulated five stages that individuals may experience, though not necessarily in a linear form, as everyone grieves in their own unique manner. These stages have been further adapted to express some of the distinctive experiences of adolescents and young adults.

- *Denial.* The teenager or young adult denies that the person close to him or her has died. "Marissa can't be dead. I just don't believe it."
- *Anger.* The teenager or young adult is angry that he or she is dying or that a loved one is deceased. "I hate my father for dying. Why did he have to leave us."
- *Bargaining.* The teenager or young adult wishes that he or she could do something different, or bargain with others or God, to evoke change regarding a terminal illness or death of a loved one. "I promise I'll help Mom out more around the house if you just make her better."
- *Depression.* The teenager or young adult feels extremely sad, may be tearful, and is consumed by intense feelings of grief. "I feel so depressed and sad all of the time about DeShawn having cancer. I don't want him to die."
- *Acceptance.* The teenager or young adult accepts the passing of a cherished loved one, and may once again begin to enjoy life. "I will always miss my dad, but I know he would want me to go to the game with my uncle and think of him. We had such great times there together."

One way to assist the bereaved in the process of grieving is through the enactment or establishment of rituals. Rituals may assist in assigning meaning to life-changing events, and they also provide a safe means and socially acceptable outlet for expressing one's emotions. Use of rituals may "symbolize continuity, stability, and the significance of personal bonds while helping people accept the inevitable change" (Walsh, 2007, p. 217).

Some rituals that may be of benefit to those who are grieving include:

- Writing a poem to the deceased loved one
- Visiting a fond place of the person who had died
- Painting or drawing about aspects of the person that are missed
- Reviewing photos of the person who has passed and reflecting on memories held of that person
- Holding a memorial service.

As previously mentioned, everyone grieves in a unique way. In addition, practitioners should remain aware of clients' emotional readiness for disclosure, as well as timing, pacing, and intensity of the therapeutic relationship. When appropriate, recalling the happy memories of those who have passed through ritual, storytelling, and artistic means may increase positive and healthy adjustment after loss (Blundell, 2001).

In the story, "I Don't Know Why She Had to Die" a young person analyzes the circumstances surrounding the serious illness and death of her best friend. Those who have suffered with this type of prolonged illness and death of a loved one may benefit from the caring support of friends, family, and professionals. Attempts to "make meaning" of the trauma and loss may also be beneficial. How to cope with such a devastating loss may also be discussed in the context of therapeutic storytelling.

In the vignette, "Life," a young person reflects on the wonderful qualities and pleasant memories shared with a loved one who has died. It also addresses the gradual adjustment process that occurs when living without a person to whom one is emotionally attached. It demonstrates that a person can cope successfully with the death of a loved one, and explores some of the mechanisms involved in this gradual process.

"That Night..." was chosen for inclusion in this book because it addresses a common cause of death among adolescents and young adults, automobile accidents. Although the death was accidental, texting while driving was involved. The story can be used to promote prevention of risky behaviors while driving, as well as serve as a springboard for discussion for those who have experienced serious car accidents.

Additional Resources

Corr, C. A., Nabe, C. M., & Corr, D. M. (2006). *Death and dying, life and living* (5th ed.). Belmont, CA: Thomson Wadsworth.

Gunaratnam, Y., & Oliviere, D. (Eds.). (2009). *Narrative and stories in health care: Illness, dying and bereavement.* New York: Oxford University Press.

Worden, J. W. (2009). *Grief counseling and grief therapy: A handbook for the mental health practitioner* (4th ed.). New York: Springer Publishing Company, LLC.

Kübler-Ross, E. (1969). *On death and dying.* New York: Macmillan.

I Don't Know Why She Had to Die

She was my best friend, and I don't know why she had to die. I used to talk to her everyday about everything that was going on in my life—and she would really listen. She actually cared about me and my family. She was there for me in the good times and the bad. We did everything together. We were best friends since second grade. Then last year she got really sick. After awhile, she became so sick that she couldn't go to school anymore and it was even hard for her to hang out with me because she was so weak and tired. We texted a lot for awhile and hung out on the Internet together though. I would go and visit her whenever I could, when she was feeling up to it.

Her illness was really horrible. Eventually, they told me that she wasn't getting better—and it crushed me. I knew it meant she was going to die. I did not know how I could live without her in my life. We had been friends for almost our entire lives and her death just devastated me. She was too young to die. Why did she have to go so early? I am so upset that she is gone, and I just feel so lonely and helpless now. What am I supposed to do without her in my life? What am I supposed to do now?

Instructions: Tell, write, or draw the answers to the following questions.

I Don't Know Why She Had to Die Questions: Level 1

1. What happened to this girl's best friend?
2. How is the girl in the story feeling?
3. Do you miss anyone in your life?
4. What could the girl in the story do to cope with the death of her best friend?
5. Who could she turn to for support?
6. How would you finish this story?

I Don't Know Why She Had to Die Questions: Level 2

1. Has anyone you know ever had a good friend die?
2. Can you tell me about what happened when his or her friend died?
3. How does this make him or her feel?
4. How did he or she cope with the death of his or her friend?
5. What is his or her story?
6. How would you change his or her story if you could?

I Don't Know Why She Had to Die Questions: Level 3

1. Have you ever had a good friend die?
2. Can you tell me about what happened when your friend died?
3. How does this make you feel?
4. How are you coping with the death of your friend?
5. What is your story?
6. How would you change your story if you could?

My Story: Level 4

Instructions: Tell, write, or draw your own story.

Coping Skills Activities

Tell, write, or draw four activities you can participate in to help you to cope positively with the death of your loved one.

Tell, write, or draw two people who you can spend time with or talk with to help you cope with the death of your loved one.

Tell, write, or draw four ways that are not helping you cope with the death of your loved one.

Life

It's been so long since she died and I still miss her so much. There is so much that I would like to tell her. I want her to know that I'm graduating from school in a week just like she wanted. She would have been so happy for me. I imagine that she would have thrown a huge party for me. I know she would have been proud of me. I miss seeing her. I miss her kind words of encouragement and caring. She was just a wonderful person. I suppose I miss just about everything about her. I am doing well though, just like she wanted me to do. I do still miss her, and I always will, but I know she wants me to be happy. And I am happy. My life is good. I graduate next week and then I'm going on an exciting trip abroad to celebrate. I can't wait to go! I love to travel. When I return I'll settle into my new life after graduation. I like to think she is looking down on me and smiling. In many ways, she is still with me.

Instructions: Tell, write, or draw the answers to the following questions.

Life Questions: Level 1

1. What is happening in this person's life?
2. How is the person in the story feeling?
3. Do you miss anyone in your life?
4. How is the person in the story coping?
5. Who could he or she turn to for support?
6. How would you finish this story?

Life Questions: Level 2

1. Has anyone you know ever had a loved one die?
2. Can you tell me about what happened when the person died?
3. How does this make him or her feel?
4. How does he or she cope with the death of his or her loved one?
5. What is his or her story?
6. How would you change his or her story if you could?

Life Questions: Level 3

1. Have you ever had a loved one die?
2. Can you tell me about what happened when your loved one died?
3. How does this make you feel?
4. How are you coping with the death of your loved one?
5. What is your story?
6. How would you change your story if you could?

My Story: Level 4

Instructions: Tell, write, or draw your own story.

That Night...

That night was just awful. I still sometimes cannot even believe that it happened. I picked Emily and Addy up so we could all go to the movies together, just like we always do. It was dark, and it started to rain. So it was kind of hard to see, and we were texting David to tell him we would be over later, after the movies. I only took the phone for a minute—I just figured it would be okay to text, especially just for a second or so. I am not even sure how it happened, but one minute we were all laughing and talking, and the next minute I lost control of the car, and we went into a spin and hit a tree.

One mistake, and now one of my best friends is dead! I will hate myself for it forever. I knew I shouldn't text and drive, but I figured that I wouldn't wreck. Things just happened so fast...

Instructions: Tell, write, or draw the answers to the following questions.

That Night Questions: Level 1

1. How is the young woman in the story feeling?
2. Why is she so upset?
3. How can this girl cope with what has happened to her and her friends?
4. How would you change this story if you could?
5. How would you finish this story?

That Night Questions: Level 2

1. Do you know anyone who has ever been in a very bad car accident?
2. Can you tell me about what happened in his or her situation?
3. How did he or she cope with what happened to him or her?
4. What did he or she learn from the accident?
5. What is his or her story?
6. How would you change his or her story if you could?

That Night Questions: Level 3

1. Have you ever been in a very bad car accident?
2. Can you tell me about what happened and how you felt?
3. Who did you turn to for help regarding what happened?

4. What are your strengths that can help you to cope with your situation?
5. What is your story?
6. How would you change your story if you could?

My Story: Level 4

Instructions: Tell, write, or draw your own story.

Poem Activity

Instructions: Write a poem in memory of your loved one who has passed away.

18

Strengths

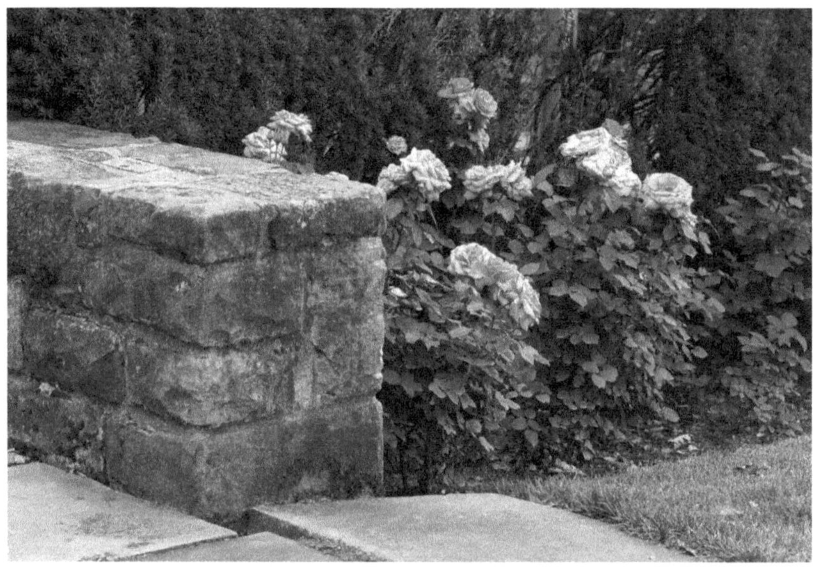

Key Practice Issues and Story Selection

The strengths perspective has emerged as one of the central tools available to practitioners and laypeople alike in their search for human potential, fulfillment, happiness, and, perhaps most important, resilience. Practitioners utilize the strengths perspective and ideas from positive psychology in the assessment of individuals, families, and communities, as well as in their repertoire of available treatment options. The strengths perspective serves as an adaptable and malleable framework that can be applied to numerous and varied life circumstances. In addition, it respects and builds upon aspects of culture and diversity.

When working with teens and young adults, it may be beneficial to shift from a pathology-based approach to a strengths-driven philosophy. Specific diagnoses may shift from being the primary focus. Instead, practitioners must search for and identify assets, gifts, and positive attributes of clients, families, and communities. However, in many circumstances, pain and hardship in individuals' lives must be valued and expressed prior to moving forward to strengths identification. Otherwise, people may feel devalued or disrespected. When the timing, pacing, and depth of therapeutic relationships are appropriate, strengths may be identified while assessing and then treating clients.

Some individual strengths to search for with adolescent and young adults include:

- Motivation to change, having a hopeful attitude, desire to improve one's self
- Intelligence, humor, athletic ability, friendliness, kindness, assertiveness, good listener, good storyteller
- Handsome, pretty, personable, easy to talk to, insightful, good friend, caring

Some strengths that families may possess include:

- Genuine concern for one another, ability to talk about problems, accepting of family members differences or imperfections
- Financial support, ability to survive despite hardship, willingness to seek help when needed
- Providing food and shelter, transportation, loving one another, providing encouragement

Some strengths to look for in the community setting include:

- A sense of belonging, providing support for members of the community
- Recreational facilities, pools, parks, and so forth
- Schools, universities, businesses, places of worship, libraries, social service agencies
- Philanthropists, foundations

All of these resources or strengths of individuals, families, and communities may be turned to or accessed in times of prosperity as well as in times of hardship. They may be built upon to improve and enhance one's quality of life. People may not view various aspects of their lives as strengths or assets, and practitioners can elicit strengths by asking appropriate questions and through using active listening and observational skills.

Some questions that Dennis Saleebey (2002) suggests using to aid in strengths identification include:

- "How have you managed to survive (or thrive) thus far, given all of the challenges you have had to contend with?"
- "What now do you want out of life?"
- "What are your hopes, visions, and aspirations?"

- "What are your special talents and abilities?"
- "What gives you genuine pleasure in life?"
- "When people say good things about you, what are they likely to say?" (p. 89)

"The Great Day" focuses on a wonderful day when everything seems to go right in a person's life. The young man in the story enjoys spending time with his friends and is excited about meeting and possibly dating a girl that he has met. This story could be used to promote positive interactions among peers when utilized with teens and young adults in treatment.

In the story "Acceptance Letter," the main character is excited and anxious while awaiting notification regarding acceptance from his university of choice. To his delight, he is accepted and has received a scholarship. This scenario could be used with students who are contemplating attending college to aid in planning and in goal setting. Also, different outcomes could be delineated which could be helpful to those contemplating alternate futures.

"The Great Workout" promotes the psychological and physical benefits of exercising and eating well. It also was included as a story in this book because it shows that a person can strive for goals and accomplish those goals. This scenario could be helpful when working with those exhibiting difficulty setting goals and who may require assistance in doing so.

In the story "Roller Coaster," friends experience a fun and exciting day together at an amusement park. It was included because it demonstrates healthy interactions among friends, and may serve as a springboard for discussion about positive friendships, relationships, and activities. In addition, it may spark conversation about how to spend relaxation and leisure time in a constructive manner.

Additional Resources

Csikszentmihalyi, M., & Csikszentmihalyi, I. S. (Eds.). (2006). *A life worth living: Contributions to positive psychology.* New York: Oxford University Press.

Freeman, E. M. (2011). *Narrative approaches in social work practice: A life span, culturally centered, strengths perspective.* Springfield, IL: Charles C. Thomas.

Helton, L. R., & Smith, M. K. (2004). *Mental health practice with children and youth: A strengths and well-being model.* Binghamton, NY: Haworth Social Work Practice Press.

Park, N., & Peterson, C. (2006). Moral competence and character strengths among adolescents: The development and validation of the Values in Action Inventory of Strengths for Youth. *Journal of Adolescence,* 29(6), 891–909.

The Great Day

I had such a great day today. It was really cool. I went to the mall with some of my friends and we just hung out. We went to some of the stores that we like and just messed around all day. While we were walking around, we met some really cute girls. I talked to a girl named Latika who goes to a different school across town, and when I get home I'm going to look her up on the Internet and friend her. I liked talking to her because she is nice, funny, and very pretty.

I think I would like to date her. Maybe I'll ask her out tonight for next weekend.

Instructions: Tell, write, or draw the answers to the following questions.

The Great Day Questions: Level 1

1. Why is this person having a great day?
2. What does this person like about the day?
3. What do you like about this person's day?
4. What did this person do right to make it a great day?
5. How would you finish this story?

The Great Day Questions: Level 2

1. Has anyone you know ever had a great day?
2. Can you tell me about what happened when he or she had a great day?
3. How does this make him or her feel?
4. What did this person do right to make it a great day?
5. What is his or her story?
6. How would you change his or her story if you wanted to?

The Great Day Questions: Level 3

1. Have you ever had a great day?
2. Can you tell me about what happened when you had a great day?
3. How does this make you feel?
4. What did you do right to make it a great day?
5. What is your story?
6. How would you change your story if you wanted to?

My Story: Level 4

Instructions: Tell, write, or draw your own story.

Acceptance Letter

Last week was Raj's interview at the university. He had been waiting to attend there all of his life. It was expected of him by his parents, and he could not disappoint them. He had worked so hard all through school, and he was hoping it would all pay off now. He had achieved excellent test scores and superior marks. Raj was waiting for the response from the university. The letter should come soon saying whether he was accepted into their program or not, and whether he would receive a scholarship.

His parents could afford to help some with tuition payments, but there was no way they could afford to pay for all of it. It was just too expensive for a family like his. The university seemed to like him and to be impressed with his academic record. "Maybe I will get in," he thought to himself.

That afternoon Raj took the train home from school and got himself an apple and some walnuts to eat. "Good brain food," he thought. Then he went back downstairs to check for the mail. It had come, and the university had sent a formal letter. He was so excited and nervous all at the same time. He went back upstairs to his apartment to open it. The news was wonderful! It read, "we are pleased to inform you that you have been accepted to our esteemed university" and "we would like to offer you a full scholarship which covers tuition and room and board." Raj could not have been more ecstatic. He felt as if his dreams were coming true, and that he could make something of his life. His parents were going to be so proud of him.

Instructions: Tell, write, or draw the answers to the following questions.

Acceptance Letter Questions: Level 1

1. What is Raj so excited about?
2. What did Raj do right to get to this point in his life?
3. What do you think that Raj wants to accomplish in his life?
4. How would you finish this story?

Acceptance Letter Questions: Level 2

1. Has anyone you know ever been very excited about his or her accomplishments?
2. What did this person do to accomplish his or her goals?
3. How does this make him or her feel?
4. What is his or her story?
5. How would you change his or her story if you wanted to?

Acceptance Letter Questions: Level 3

1. Have you ever accomplished something that you were very proud of?
2. Can you tell me about what you accomplished?
3. What did you have to do to accomplish your goal?
4. How does this make you feel?
5. What is your story?
6. How would you change your story if you wanted to?

My Story: Level 4

Instructions: Tell, write, or draw your own story.

The Great Workout

Man, I had the best workout today. I lifted for awhile and felt so pumped up afterward. Then I went for a run and went one mile past my goal. I got that high feeling that comes after a good run. There's just nothing quite like it.

I'm eating right too, a lot of vegetables and lean protein. Sometimes I make low-fat, low-sugar fruit smoothies with strawberries, bananas, and blueberries. They taste awesome and keep me in top shape. This should help me keep weight and develop more lean muscle mass, which I need.

If I keep training like this, I'll definitely be ready for the competition that's coming up. I want to win so badly I can feel it in my bones.

Instructions: Tell, write, or draw the answers to the following questions.

The Great Workout Questions: Level 1

1. Why is this person feeling so good?
2. What does this person like about the day?
3. What goal is this person working toward?
4. What is this person doing right in his or her life?
5. How would you finish this story?

The Great Workout Questions: Level 2

1. Has anyone you know ever felt really good about an activity or hobby that he or she participates in?
2. Can you tell me what he or she likes about the activity or hobby?
3. Does he or she ever set goals to strive toward to improve his or her skills?
4. What is his or her story?
5. How would you change his or her story if you wanted to?

The Great Workout Questions: Level 3

1. Have you ever felt really good about an activity or hobby that you participate in?
2. Can you tell me what you like about the activity or hobby?
3. Do you ever set goals to strive toward to improve your skills?
4. What is your story?
5. How would you change your story if you wanted to?

My Story: Level 4

Instructions: Tell, write, or draw your own story.

Roller Coaster by Ashley Slivinske

A rush of adrenaline sped through my veins. My piercing blue eyes stared like a deer in headlights as the green light flickered on.

"It's time to go," I shouted to Emily. The roller coaster went from zero to 120 miles per hour. The only thing I could hear was the loud pounding in my chest. The only thing I could feel was the lump in my throat. At that moment, nothing else in the world mattered.

It shot like a rocket 180 degrees skyward. At the peak, the moment was serene, but then we shot down. Neither of us spoke. We glanced at each other, trembling yet smiling. If we can do this, you can do anything.

Instructions: Tell, write, or draw the answers to the following questions.

Roller Coaster Questions: Level 1

1. Why is this person feeling so happy and excited?
2. What does this person like about the day?
3. What kind of personality does this person have?
4. What is this person doing right in his or her life?
5. How would you finish this story?

Roller Coaster Questions: Level 2

1. Do you know a person who enjoys fun activities?
2. Can you tell me what activities he or she enjoys?
3. What kind of personality does this person have?
4. What is this person doing right in his or her life?
5. What is his or her story?
6. How would you change his or her story if you wanted to?
7. How would you finish this story?

Roller Coaster Questions: Level 3

1. Do you enjoy fun activities?
2. Can you tell me what activities you enjoy?
3. What kind of personality do you have?
4. What are you doing right in your life?
5. What is your story?
6. How would you change your story if you wanted to?
7. How would you finish this story?

My Story: Level 4

Instructions: Tell, write, or draw your own story.

Strengths Activity: The PLAN Method of Intervention

Instructions: Tell, write, or draw the answers to the following questions or statements.

Positive action creates positive lifestyles

What are some positive actions you can take in your life?

Look to the future

What do you want to accomplish in the future?

Activate your strengths, inside and out

What are some of your strengths?

Never give up on yourself

When I feel like quitting or giving up I will…

Activity: Positive Action Creates Positive Change

Instructions: Using the diagram below, tell, write or draw the actions you can take to improve your life.

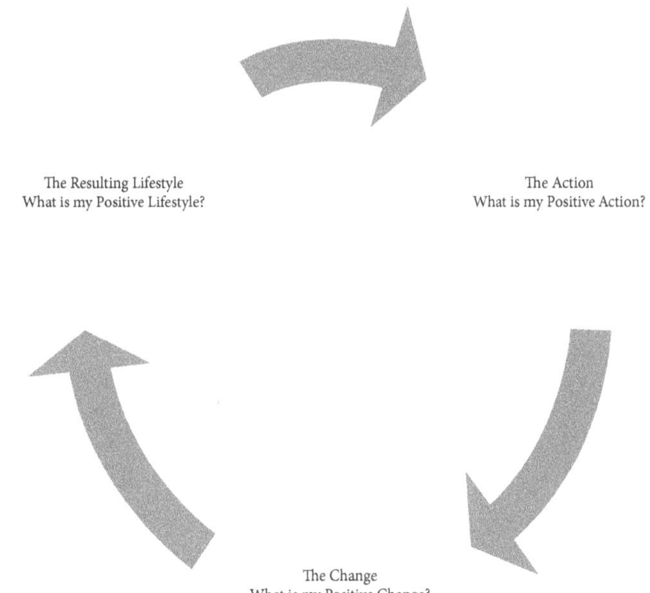

Strengths Activity: Look to the Future

Instructions: Tell, write, or draw the answers to the following statements to help you to look toward the future. With the help of your friend, parent, or therapist, make a plan to accomplish your goals. Set the plan into action, if you desire.

Tomorrow I would like to . . .
One week from now I would like to . . .
One month from now I would like to . . .
Six months from now I would like to . . .
One year from now I would like to . . .
Two years from now I would like to . . .
Five years from now I would like to . . .
Ten years from now I would like to . . .
Twenty years from now I would like to . . .

Strengths Activity: My Plan Leads to My Future

Instructions: Based upon the previous activity "Look to the Future," choose a time period and set goals to work toward your plans for the future. Tell, write, or draw how you plan to work toward your goals.

Example:

Goal ⇨ Two years from now, I would like to attend college. My goal to work toward this is to research five different colleges on the Internet, and to figure out how I need to apply for school and how to apply for financial aid.

Goal ⇨

Goal ⇨

Writing Activity

Instructions: Free write about the following. There is no right or wrong answer.

Who am I?

Who am I becoming?

Thinking Outside the Box about Yourself Activity

Instructions: Tell, write, or draw, outside of the box provided, as many unique, quirky, fun, and positive qualities about yourself as you can.

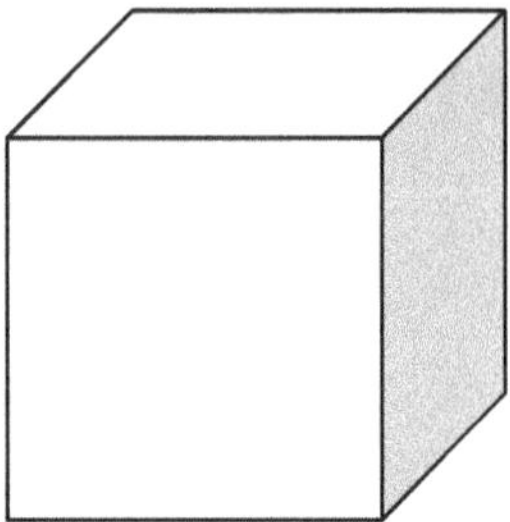

Strengths and Areas Needing Growth in Your Community Questions

Instructions: Tell, write, or draw the answers to the following questions.

1. What are some positive aspects of your community?
2. What activities would you like to participate in or organizations would you like to join in your community? (e.g. health clubs, gyms, social organizations, religious groups, and so forth).
3. What aspects of your community need to be improved?
4. How could someone or an organization begin to move toward positive change in your community?

Create a Video Game Activity

Instructions: Create the plot and characters for a video game that you would like to be a character in. You may be yourself, or have another character stand for you. Be creative and have fun!

19

Community Violence and Gangs

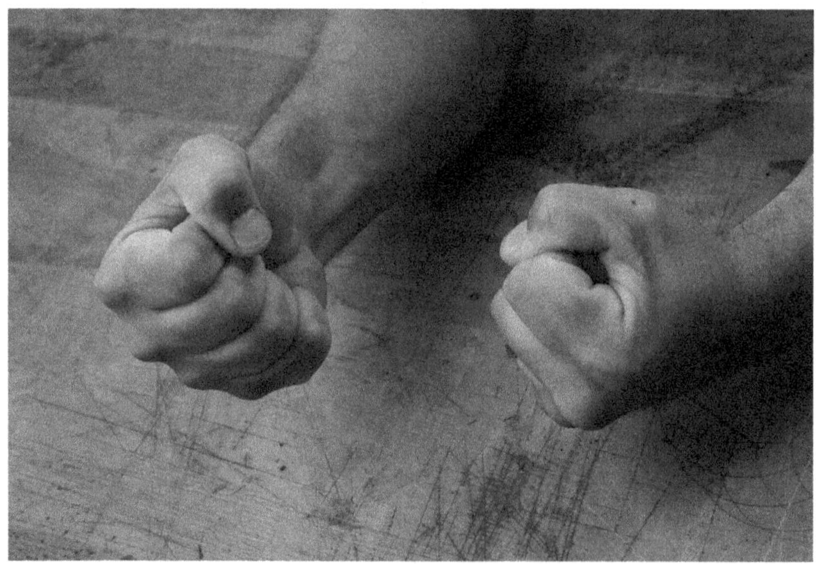

Key Practice Issues and Story Selection

Community violence is an issue that affects many different cross sections of society. Although the family is the major source of socialization for adolescents and young adults, the community and peer group within the context of particular neighborhoods and communities affects both positive and negative development. Many living in neighborhoods where the crime rate is high will become victims of crime.

Others will be negatively influenced into partaking in risk-taking, violent behaviors that may result in serious injury and death to self and others. Incarceration of adolescents and young adults often results. In turn, these adolescents and young adults become absent fathers and mothers, leaving their own children to be raised with the often cumulative disadvantage of having an incarcerated parent, poverty, and exposure to substance abuse and violence.

Types of violence affecting our youth and young adults include assaults, robberies, and rapes. Those between the ages of 12 to 19 are two to three times more likely to be victims of the aforementioned crimes than adults in general (Ashford & LeCroy, 2010). Shootings and stabbings involving drugs and gang violence are also unfortunately common in certain neighborhoods. They disproportionately occur in many urban areas where crime, poverty, and drug abuse are prevalent. However, gun violence and other types of violence can and does occur in nearly every type of community, including suburban and rural neighborhoods.

Adolescents and young adults may benefit from assistance in the following areas:

- Supportive counseling should be provided for the overwhelming grief, loss, and trauma incurred and suffered as a victim of crime, or multiple losses of friends and family members due to violence.
- Interventions promoting peaceful mediation instead of violent actions should be taught.
- Promotion of hope and planning for fulfillment of dreams that may seem impossible or difficult to achieve when faced with frequent community violence, poverty, and hopelessness.
- Planning for college for those whose families are not familiar with the college admissions and financial aid process.
- Planning and practicing employment skills such as completing job applications, writing resumes, and dressing appropriately for work in order to encourage positive alternatives to violence and illegal activities.
- Advocating at the community, state, national, and global level for increased support for families living in high crime areas.

The vignette "I Saw Them All Get Shot," describes a scenario of a gunman shooting innocent victims and the ensuing trauma. Symptoms of post-traumatic stress are portrayed, and the emotions of shock, disbelief, and fear expressed. Other emotions involving anger, distress and helplessness may be explored in a therapeutic setting. It is hoped that clients who have experienced this type of violent trauma will be able to find calm, peace, empowerment and regain a sense of safety and control as they progress through their healing journeys.

The story "I Got Shot," addresses the complicated situation and emotions surrounding a young person who has directly been a victim of community violence. Those who have been victims of violence may relate to this scenario, and may benefit from retelling their own stories in a safe and supportive environment. Strengths and coping mechanisms may be built upon to encourage the fostering of resilience.

"My Brothers" is applicable for use with individuals who may be vulnerable to joining gangs in order to discuss positive life alternatives besides gangs and violence. Also, those entrenched in gang or street life may identify with the circumstances portrayed in this vignette. Hopefully, with much support they may be encouraged to examine other ways of living that promote healthy, non-violent interactions.

Additional Resources

Briere, J. N., & Lanktree, C. B. (2012). *Treating complex trauma in adolescents and young adults.* Thousand Oaks, CA: Sage.

Burnell, J. (2013). Small change: Understanding cultural action as a resource for unlocking assets and building resilience in communities. *Community Development Journal,* 48(1), 134–150.

Cooley-Strickland, M., Quille, T. J., Griffin, R. S., Stuart, E. A., Bradshaw, C. P., & Furr-Holden, D. (2009). Community violence and youth: Affect, behavior, substance use, and academics. *Clinical Child and Family Psychology Review,* 12(2), 127–156. doi: 10.1007/s10567-009-0051-6

Delgado, M. (2000). *Community social work practice in an urban context: The potential of a capacity-enhancement perspective.* New York: Oxford University Press.

I Saw Them All Get Shot

My God, it was just so horrible when it happened. I couldn't even believe it was happening. We were just minding our own business and going about our day when he walked right in with a gun. He started pointing it and firing. It all happened so fast, but it was just so terrifying. Before I even had time to process what had happened, several people were lying on the ground, injured or dead. I could not believe my eyes and ears. It all seemed so unreal. How am I going to recover from this? I never wanted anything like this to happen. I try not to think about it, but sometimes it just pops into my head when I don't want to think about it. Now sometimes I have graphic nightmares about that day, and they just feel so real. I wake up sweating sometimes too. If I am out shopping with my friends and I hear a loud noise, I just jump and feel very afraid because I think that someone is shooting again. I really just want to feel better again. I want to feel safe and normal.

Instructions: Tell, write, or draw the answers to the following questions.

I Saw Them All Get Shot Questions: Level 1

1. What did this person witness?
2. How does he or she feel about what happened?
3. What would you tell this person to help him or her?
4. What can he or she do to cope with the situation?
5. What are this person's strengths?
6. How would you finish this story?

I Saw Them All Get Shot Questions: Level 2

1. Has anyone you know been affected by violence or a shooting?
2. Can you tell me about what happened to him or her?
3. How does this make him or her feel?
4. How does he or she cope with the violence that occurred?
5. What is his or her story?
6. How would you change his or her story if you could?

I Saw Them All Get Shot Questions: Level 3

1. Have you ever witnessed a shooting or violence?
2. Can you tell me what happened?
3. How does this make you feel?
4. What are your strengths that help you to cope with the shooting or violence?
5. What is your story?
6. How would you change your story if you could?

My Story: Level 4

Instructions: Tell, write, or draw your own story.

I Got Shot

It was so freaking scary and unreal that night when I got shot. Everybody was just hanging out outside and then Terrell and Trey started getting really mad. I don't even know what they started fighting about. Terrell pushed Trey and before I knew what was really happening, Trey pulled out his gun and bullets were flying everywhere. It was so stupid.

It all happened so quickly. Before I knew what was even happening, Terrell was laying there on the ground with everybody hovering around him. I guess I am lucky—I only got caught in the crossfire. I was shot in the arm. It could have been a lot worse . . .

Instructions: Tell, write, or draw the answers to the following questions.

I Got Shot Questions: Level 1

1. What happened to this young man?
2. How does he feel about what happened?
3. What is happening in his neighborhood?
4. What can he do to prevent and avoid the violence?
5. What are this young man's strengths?
6. How would you finish this story?

I Got Shot Questions: Level 2

1. Has anyone you know been affected by violence such as shootings in his or her neighborhood?
2. Can you tell me about what happened to him or her?
3. How does this make him or her feel?
4. How does he or she cope with the neighborhood violence?
5. What is his or her story?
6. How would you change his or her story if you could?

I Got Shot Questions: Level 3

1. Do you know anyone close to you who has been shot?
2. Can you tell me what happened when he or she was shot?
3. How does this make you feel?
4. What are your strengths that help you to cope with the shooting?
5. What is your story?
6. How would you change your story if you could?

My Story: Level 4

Instructions: Tell, write, or draw your own story.

My Brothers

They're my brothers and I won't let them down. I do for them, because they do for me. They've got my back—and I've got theirs. I'll do whatever it takes. I'm ready to defend our territory. I've passed the initiation; I've proven what kind of man I am. Now I am ready.

They shot my brother, and now it's time for payback. No more waiting, no more messing around. Revenge is sweet.

Instructions: Tell, write, or draw the answers to the following questions.

My Brothers Questions: Level 1

1. What happened to this young man's brother?
2. How does he feel about what happened?
3. What is happening in this young man's neighborhood?
4. Do you think this young man is in a gang?
5. What will happen if he seeks revenge?
6. How would you finish this story?

My Brothers Questions: Level 2

1. Has anyone you know ever been in a gang or involved in neighborhood violence?
2. Can you tell me about what happened to him or her?
3. How does this make him or her feel?
4. Did he or she ever leave the gang or stop his or her involvement in community violence?
5. What is his or her story?
6. How would you change his or her story if you could?

My Brothers Questions: Level 3

1. Have you ever been in a gang or involved in community violence?
2. Can you tell me what this experience was like for you?
3. How does this make you feel?
4. Did you ever leave the gang or stop your involvement in community violence?
5. What are your strengths that could help you to stop your involvement with the gang and community violence?
6. What is your story?
7. How would you change your story if you could?

My Story: Level 4

Instructions: Tell, write, or draw your own story.

20

Independence

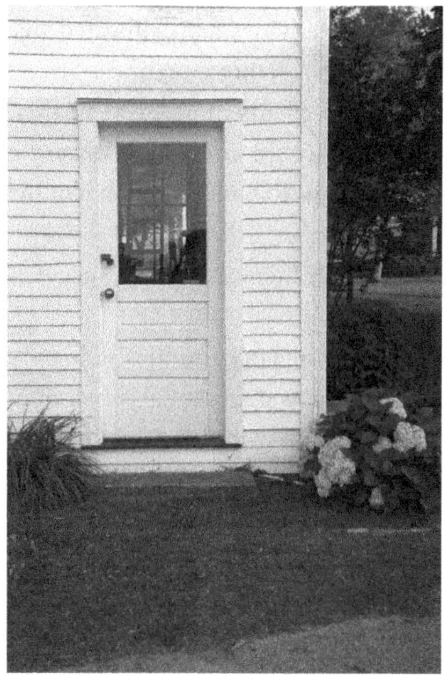

Key Practice Issues and Story Selection

A large part of emotional and psychological growth during adolescence involves the development of identity while during young adulthood, one's identity becomes further entrenched or solidified. As one continues to mature as a young adult, it is natural and typical for a person to desire increased independence. One way to express this wish is through breaking away psychologically and literally from one's parents.

This breaking away process may involve spending more frequent and intimate time spent with peers and romantic interests, delving into school activities and work, as well as the eventual desire to leave the home of one's parents. Many will choose to set up an apartment or home independently or with a roommate, cohabitate, or marry. This may be difficult for some adolescents who are unprepared to live on their own. Tasks which must be mastered in order to successfully achieve independence include: the ability to earn and manage money and financial responsibilities, the knowledge of how to grocery shop and cook, the maturity and diligence to maintain a decently clean living environment, and the ability to care for one's self, and sometimes others (e.g. spouses, children) (Matto, 2003).

The readiness to apply these skills will vary markedly from person to person based on maturity level, knowledge and practice provided by parents and schools regarding real-world preparedness, and so forth. Independent living skills may be more difficult to master for certain groups of people who may lack the availability of long-term financial, emotional, and social supports. Those with various mental or physical disabilities, and those leaving foster care, group homes, or residential treatment facilities could likely benefit from additional emotional, financial and community supports.

In this section of the book, activities are delineated that allow for exploration of readiness to move into independent living situations. Strengths and weaknesses may be explored with practitioners and clients in order to further develop skill areas needing improvement. Hopefully this would contribute toward enhanced confidence and self-sufficiency in the real world. Tips to build independent living preparedness include:

- Arrange for a meeting with a peer mentor who has successfully achieved independence.
- Arrange for possible job shadowing opportunities so high school aged students and young adults can experience aspects of potential career opportunities.
- Assist the adolescent or young adult with the preparation of a résumé or job application.
- Practice interviewing skills such as shaking hands, maintaining eye contact, and appropriate use of language.
- If facilities are available, practice or teach real world skills such as cooking, cleaning, grocery shopping, and financial planning.
- Make a list of contacts for the person to call or text if he or she needs guidance or additional assistance.

In the story "My First Job," a young person is excited yet nervous about starting a new position. He or she is preparing and practicing how to interact with coworkers and superiors in the first days of a new job. Also, the character is gaining valuable insight and recommendations from parents and an older sibling. This scenario could be beneficial to any young adult entering the workforce, to reinforce positive work-related behaviors leading toward career success.

"Moving Out" is a vignette that explores the difficulties encountered by a young adult who desires to leave his or her parents' home, but is unsure how to accomplish this goal. If clients identify with this story, they likely could benefit from guidance and direction regarding identification of goals and goal setting. How to turn their desires into reality could be examined and planned, with the help of a caring professional.

In the scenario "The Interview," a young adult practices and plans for an important job interview. This scene could assist teens and young adults in the job interview preparation process. Those who are unfamiliar could benefit from learning how to prepare. Those who are familiar with the interview process could benefit from additional practice and assistance with relaxation prior to an interview.

Additional Resources

Clark, H. B., Koroloff, N., Geller, J., & Sondheimer, D. L. (2008). Research on transition to adulthood: Building the evidence base to inform services and supports for youth and young adults with serious mental health disorders. *Journal of Behavioral Health Services & Research*, 35(4), 365–372.

Hendry, L. B., & Kloep, M. (2012). *Adolescence and adulthood: Transitions and transformations.* New York: Palgrave Macmillan.

Rosenberg, L. (2008). Building a meaningful future for young people with mental illness. *Journal of Behavioral Health Services & Research*, 35(4), 362–364.

Sachs, B. (2013). *Family-centered treatment with struggling young adults: A clinician's guide to the transition from adolescence to autonomy.* New York: Routledge.

My First Job

Tomorrow I start my first real job, and I'm so excited. I'm really nervous too. I have the perfect outfit picked out to wear. I will look professional yet friendly. My mom and my best friend told me to be myself and to be friendly, yet professional, to everyone. I have been practicing my handshake with my father. My dad said that I will probably meet a lot of people on the first day, so I will have to try to remember people's names. Then I will meet with Human Resources to discuss my new position, company policies, and to complete several forms that are required. Then I will likely receive training and instructions about what to do in my position. I hope I can learn everything quickly so that I will be successful. I think I can do it. My older sister told me that it is important to be a team player, so that people will want to work with me. I can't wait to get started with the company, and I can't believe that I landed this job!

Instructions: Tell, write, or draw the answers to the following questions.

My First Job Questions: Level 1

1. How does this young man or woman feel about his or her first job?
2. Do you think he or she will do well?
3. What are some positive steps he or she has taken to make the first day on the job a success?
4. What are some strengths that he or she could build on to improve his or her chances of succeeding on the job?
5. How would you finish this story?

My First Job Questions: Level 2

1. Has anyone you know ever prepared for and gone for a first job?
2. Did he or she do well on the job?
3. How does this make him or her feel?
4. What helped him or her to prepare for his or her first job?
5. What are some strengths that he or she could build on to improve his or her job skills?
6. What is his or her story?
7. How would you change his or her story if you could?

My First Job Questions: Level 3

1. Have you ever gone for or prepared for a first day on a job?
2. Did you do well?
3. How did this make you feel?
4. What are some possible options available to you to prepare for your next job?
5. What are some strengths that you could build on to improve your job skills?
6. What is your story?
7. How would you change your story if you could?

My Story: Level 4

Instructions: Tell, write, or draw your own story.

Moving Out

I feel like such a screw up. I'd like to move out of my parents' house, but I don't know how. I think my parents want me to go—but I'm just kind of stuck. I never went to college, and my job is just okay. What am I going to do? I feel like I don't have any options. If I do have any, I guess I'm not sure what they are.

Instructions: Tell, write, or draw the answers to the following questions.

Moving Out Questions: Level 1

1. How does this young man or woman feel about still living at home?
2. Do you think he or she can move out of his or her parents' house?
3. What are some possible options available to him or her?
4. What are some strengths that he or she could build on to improve his or her life?
5. How would you finish this story?

Moving Out Questions: Level 2

1. Does anyone you know still live at home with his or her parents?
2. Do you think he or she wants to move out of his or her parents' house?
3. How does this make him or her feel?
4. What are some possible options available to him or her?
5. What are some strengths that he or she could build on to improve his or her life?
6. What is his or her story?
7. How would you change his or her story if you could?

Moving Out Questions: Level 3

1. Do you still live at home with your parents?
2. Do you want to move out of your parents' house?
3. How does this make you feel?
4. What are some possible options available to you?
5. What are some strengths that you could build on to improve your life?
6. What is your story?
7. How would you change your story if you could?

My Story: Level 4

Instructions: Tell, write, or draw your own story.

The Interview

I have my first real interview tomorrow, and I'm really nervous. I have been practicing answering interview questions with my friends, and I think I will do okay. I researched the company, and I feel like I know a lot about them. I've been practicing my handshake too. I know that I have to remember to completely shut off my cell phone during the interview so it doesn't ring or vibrate! That would be so embarrassing, and I probably wouldn't get the job if that happened.

I have one of my nicest outfits picked out and I feel pretty confident that I am qualified for the position. Hopefully nothing will come up about that old picture of me at the party on my site that I took down, but if it does, I know how to explain it to the employer.

I really hope I get the job!

Instructions: Tell, write, or draw the answers to the following questions.

The Interview Questions: Level 1

1. How does this young man or woman feel about his or her interview?
2. Do you think he or she will do well?
3. What are some positive steps he or she has taken to make the interview a success?
4. What are some strengths that he or she could build on to improve his or her chances of getting the job?
5. How would you finish this story?

The Interview Questions: Level 2

1. Has anyone you know ever prepared for and gone for a job interview?
2. Did he or she do well on the interview?
3. How did this make him or her feel?
4. What are some possible options available to him or her to prepare for his or her next job interview?
5. What are some strengths that he or she could build on to improve his or her job skills?
6. What is his or her story?
7. How would you change his or her story if you could?

The Interview Questions: Level 3

1. Have you ever gone for or prepared for a job interview?
2. Did you do well on the interview?
3. How did this make you feel?
4. What are some possible options available to you to prepare for your next job interview?
5. What are some strengths that you could build on to improve your job skills?
6. What is your story?
7. How would you change your story if you could?

My Story: Level 4

Instructions: Tell, write, or draw your own story.

What are My Options?

Instructions: Tell, write, or draw the answers to the following questions.

Is attending college an option?
Is taking a training course an option?
Is getting a better job an option?
Is getting an apartment with or without a roommate an option?
Is moving to a new city or state an option?

Moving Out Questions

What do I need when I move out and set up my own apartment?
Where can I get the items I need?
Who could I count on to help me?
Who could I count on for support if I get into trouble?
How can I manage my money?
How can I learn to cook and do laundry (if I don't already know how)?

Where Am I? Activity Sheet

Instructions: In the center circle, tell, write, or draw where you would like to be in the future. In the outer circles, tell, write, or draw what you need to do to get to where you would like to be in the future.

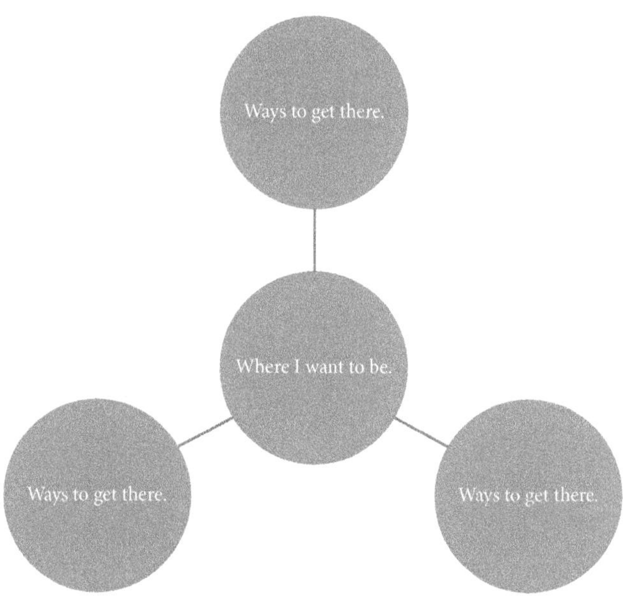

21

Cultural and Religious Issues

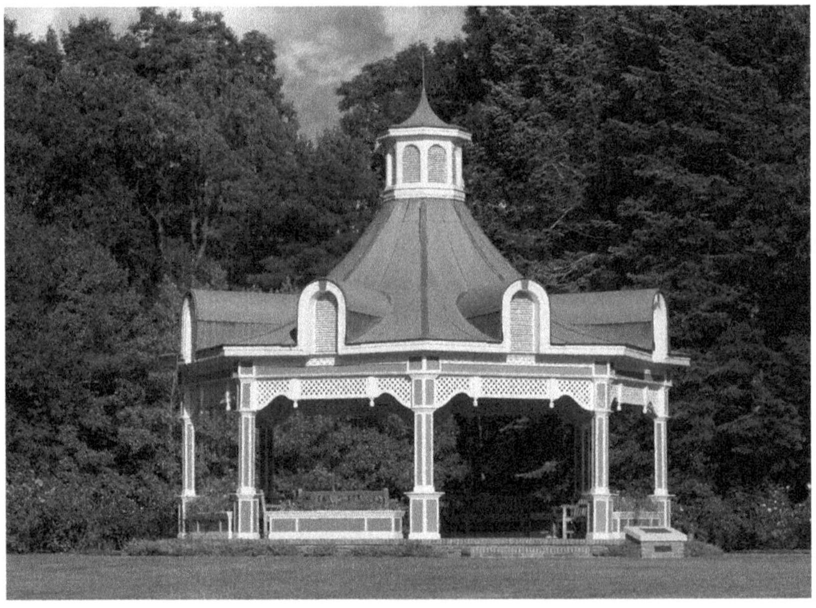

Key Practice Issues and Story Selection

Examining the culture in which adolescents and young adults are raised enables therapists to gain insight into their system of beliefs, values, and behavior. Cultural aspects of family, communities, and societies have a powerful influence on the development of youth. Adolescents and young adults are experiencing spurts in growth, changes in hormones, sexual maturity, as well as neurological changes which influence impulse control. This period of development for some has been described as a period of physical and emotional turmoil, and is embedded in a cultural context. Youth are in the process of becoming adults but often lack the necessary psychological maturity, social status, and financial resources to function responsibly and independently in their society (Chen & Farruggia, 2002).

Often during this time, individuals experience an increased level of incidence in depression, delinquency, and drug and alcohol use. Some also have psychosomatic complaints such as headaches, stomachaches, and sleeping difficulties; problems regarding self-esteem; and eating disorders to name a few (Schulenberg & Maggs, 1997). Perspectives regarding many of these developmental, psychological, and health challenges are culturally grounded. During the trying time of adjusting to bodily and mental changes and increases in social responsibility, it may be necessary to have someone to talk to regarding these important issues. Understanding clients' cultural frameworks enables practitioners to better meet their needs and to increase the effectiveness of treatment.

Religion has been found in many cultures to be an important part of this developmental process also. Traditions are passed down which help teens and young adults develop a sense of belonging, morality, and social responsibility. Religious codes of conduct can provide guidelines for behaving which discourages violating the social order. Religious youth are thought to be more integrated into society, are more likely to help people in need and engage in community service, and are more likely to avoid self-destructive and delinquent behaviors (Lerner, Jacobs, & Wertlieb, 2003). However, in this period of development, individuals often question what their parents, guardians, teachers, and religious leaders teach them in their quest to understand themselves and their place in society. During this transition from adolescence to adulthood it is often a time to seek the advice and counsel of an experienced therapist, religious leader, or mentor.

Cultural and religious differences impact numerous teens and young adults in the United States and throughout the world today. These differences affect the developing person in a multitude of ways, including amplifying any pre-existing feelings of differentness or of "not fitting in," that in many instances are already normative for many teens and young adults. Issues involving ethnic, gender, sexual orientation, and racial relationships and probable ensuing conflicts may complicate the identity confusion that adolescents attempt to surmount. Building intimacy in close relationships with friends and romantic partners may be strained when societal influences regarding cultural and religious expectations are involved.

Additionally those individuals who already live with challenges such as depression, anxiety, and other disorders may be at an increased risk for complications and discrimination based on double or triple minority status. For example, if a young adult is an African American female who is also a lesbian, she is much more likely to incur harassment, prejudice, and discrimination based on matters related to culture, gender, and sexual orientation. Another instance would be discrimination against an Asian male who uses a wheelchair.

In recent years, attention has been brought to the forefront regarding bullying and sexual orientation. Adolescents who are gay, bisexual, lesbian, questioning, or transgendered continue to be harassed and discriminated against, sometimes to the point of personal despair. Teens and young adults in these groups as well as other cultural, racial, gender and religious groups may at times be unable to cope with harassment, persecution and bullying, which sometimes contributes to a person committing suicide. Mental health professionals and others must attempt to foster inclusion and acceptance of those suffering from bullying, and advocate for positive change in society.

However, through positive support and the use of strengths-based interventions designed to magnify the many positive aspects of one's culture or religion, it is possible to overcome difficulties or misunderstandings based on these points. At times, bridges of understanding may be crossed by explaining truths and dispelling myths regarding animosity and prejudice that may be hurtful, destructive, and damaging to non-dominant groups. Ways of managing, coping, and handling oppression may foster resilience in those faced with these challenging circumstances. In addition, the power of advocacy, political activism and support for marginalized individuals, families, groups, organizations, and communities should not be underestimated.

The first vignette, "My Roommates" is an example of a group of diverse individuals who upon first introduction, were somewhat leery of one another based on religious and cultural differences. However, as they grew as individuals and were able to relate to one another on a personal level, they found that they not only tolerated one another, but actually became friends. It is a positive portrayal of healthy diversity in action. This story could be utilized therapeutically to show how people who are very different can still co-exist in a healthy, positive, and mutually enjoyable manner.

"They Don't Understand Our Way of Life," was included in this section because it addresses the complex relationships between two groups of people who feel they are very different from one another. This story could be used to bridge the gap of misunderstanding between multiple groups of people throughout the world. It is hoped that commonalities could be found that could foster and promote peaceful understanding and compromise between differing cultural and religious groups.

The story, "They Call Me a Terrorist" addresses current and relevant issues regarding prejudice, hate and discrimination. Historically, and yet today, in times of international conflict and war, innocent people are sometimes mislabeled, discriminated against or harassed. This story is designed to enable a person to further develop existing coping mechanisms in order to surmount such difficult circumstances.

Additional Resources

Arnett, J. J. (2013). *Adolescence and emerging adulthood: A cultural approach* (5th ed.). Boston, MA: Pearson.

Johnson, W. E. (2010). *Social work with African American males: Health, mental health, and social policy.* New York: Oxford University Press.

Josselson, R., & Harway, M. (Eds.). (2012). *Navigating multiple identities: Race, gender, culture, nationality, and roles.* New York: Oxford University Press.

Rockenbach, A. B., & Mayhem, M. J. (Eds.). (2013). *Spirituality in college students' lives: Translating research into practice.* New York: Routledge.

My Roommates

My roommates couldn't have been more different, particularly regarding religious beliefs. One of my roommates was an atheist, one was Jewish, and the other was Muslim. I myself was raised as a Christian. At first we all were standoffish with each other because of what we had been taught as children. Over the months we became friends and finally were comfortable enough to talk about our religions or lack thereof and what each of us believed. We decided to go with each other to our respective mosques, synagogues, and churches to experience the others' religions. We actually could do this as their respective, main days of worship were Fridays, Saturdays, and Sundays. Even our roommate who didn't have any experience with religion said he would go just to see what we had all been talking about. We talked about the differences, but soon learned of the similarities. Some of our elders were not too happy with what we were doing, but we still saw the good things in each of our religions and each other. We now have decided to learn more about some other religions such as Hinduism, Buddhism, Shinto, Taoism, among others.

Instructions: Tell, write, or draw the answers to the following questions.

My Roommates Questions: Level 1

1. How does this young man or woman feel about friends with different belief systems?
2. How do you think the diverse people in the story were able to get along so well?
3. What are some differences and similarities among them?
4. What are some positive personal qualities of the people in the story?
5. How would you finish this story?

My Roommates Questions: Level 2

1. Has anyone you know ever had friends who had different cultural or religious beliefs?
2. How were the diverse friends able to get along?
3. What were some differences and similarities among them?
4. What are some of their positive personal qualities?
5. What is his or her story?
6. How would you change his or her story if you could?

My Roommates Questions: Level 3

1. Have you ever felt misunderstood or understood because of your culture or religion?
2. How does this make you feel?
3. How do you cope with feeling misunderstood by others?
4. What are some positive ways that you could handle being misunderstood?
5. What are some strengths that you use to foster understanding of your culture or religion?
6. What is your story?
7. How would you change your story if you could?

My Story: Level 4

Instructions: Tell, write, or draw your own story.

They Don't Understand Our Way of Life

I suppose our way of life is different from other people. Sometimes I feel like they don't really understand us. I suppose that sometimes I feel like I don't really understand them. It is like we are worlds apart, even though we just live about a half mile down the road from each other. We certainly act differently than they do. We even look different too.

I know we are all human beings, but I don't know what we even have in common with them. I suppose there must be similarities.

Instructions: Tell, write, or draw the answers to the following questions.

They Don't Understand Our Way of Life Questions: Level 1

1. How does this young man or woman feel about being misunderstood?
2. Who do you think the two groups of people in the story represent?
3. What are some differences and similarities among the two groups of people?
4. Do you think the two groups of people get along with each other?
5. How would you finish this story?

They Don't Understand Our Way of Life Questions: Level 2

1. Has anyone you know ever felt misunderstood because of his or her culture or religion?
2. How does this make him or her feel?
3. How did he or she cope with feeling misunderstood by others?
4. What are some other ways that he or she could handle being misunderstood?
5. What are some strengths that he or she could build on to improve his or her coping skills?
6. What is his or her story?
7. How would you change his or her story if you could?

They Don't Understand Our Way of Life Questions: Level 3

1. Have you ever felt misunderstood because of your culture or religion?
2. How does this make you feel?
3. How do you cope with feeling misunderstood by others?
4. What are some other ways that you could handle being misunderstood?
5. What are some strengths that you could build on to improve your coping skills?
6. What is your story?
7. How would you change your story if you could?

My Story: Level 4

Instructions: Tell, write, or draw your own story.

They Call Me a Terrorist

Hate breeds hate, that's what they say. Well I feel like I hate them—because they call me a terrorist. Well, I'll tell you this; I am not a terrorist. I never have been and I never will be. I don't like the terrorists anymore than they do. I think that what they do is horrible.

I wish the people who call me that would just leave me alone. I have never hurt anyone, and I don't intend to in the future. I wish there were no terrorists, and I wish that everyone was peaceful. This world is really screwed up.

Instructions: Tell, write, or draw the answers to the following questions.

They Call Me a Terrorist Questions: Level 1

1. How is this young man or woman feeling?
2. Why do you think people in the story are calling him a terrorist?
3. What are some ways this person could cope positively with the situation?
4. How would you finish this story?

They Call Me a Terrorist Questions: Level 2

1. Has anyone you know ever felt misunderstood or mislabeled because of his or her culture or religion?
2. How does this make him or her feel?
3. How did he or she cope with feeling misunderstood by others?
4. What are some other ways that he or she could handle being misunderstood or mislabeled?
5. What are some strengths that he or she could build on to improve his or her coping skills?
6. What is his or her story?
7. How would you change his or her story if you could?

They Call Me a Terrorist Questions: Level 3

1. Have you ever felt misunderstood or mislabeled because of your culture or religion?
2. How does this make you feel?
3. How do you cope with feeling misunderstood or mislabeled by others?
4. What are some other ways that you could handle being misunderstood or mislabeled?
5. What are some strengths that you could build on to improve your coping skills?
6. What is your story?
7. How would you change your story if you could?

My Story: Level 4

Instructions: Tell, write, or draw your own story.

22

Job Loss and Poverty

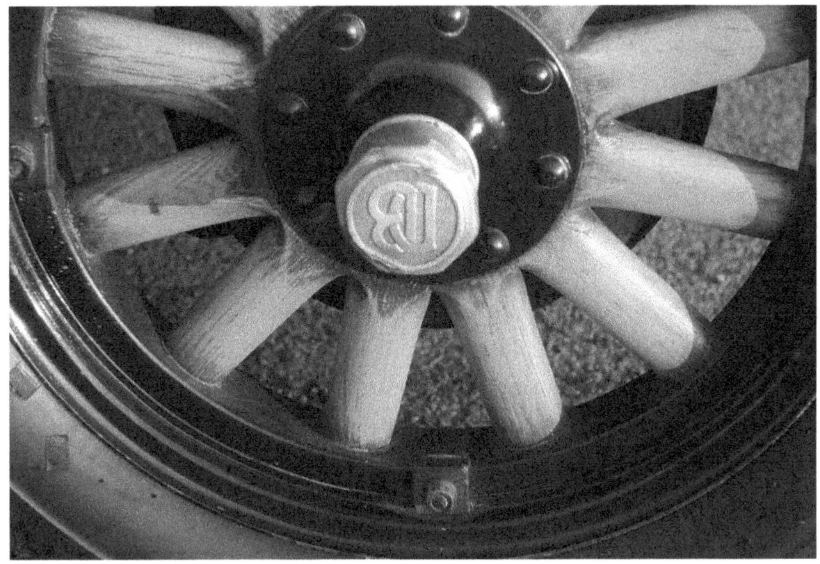

Key Practice Issues and Story Selection

One way to examine the meaning of the word poverty is by exploration of its definition. One way to think of poverty is as "the extent to which a person does without resources" (De Vol, 2006). Resources that literally may be lacking from a person's life include basic needs such as clean water, food, clothing, housing, and so forth. In addition, more figurative resources may also be missing, such as a lack of safe and well-paying jobs or career opportunities, inadequate social supports to assist with family functioning, lack of excellent educational opportunities, neighborhoods that possess higher levels of crime and decreased feelings of safety, and less opportunity to engage in healthy leisure and recreational activities within one's own neighborhood or community.

The economic environment in which one grows and develops affects aspects of both current and future human development. In today's economic climate, adolescents and young adults may find themselves competing with much older and more qualified individuals for lower paying employment opportunities. This may create added difficulties for them related to acquiring gainful employment and to flourishing economically as independent young adults. In turn, these events may potentially hinder further development in other areas such as attaining educational and relationship goals (e.g. obtaining a college degree or marriage).

However, steps may be taken to assist individuals by examining all possible opportunities that may exist to help people to overcome financial and economic barriers. These opportunities and challenges could take the form of investing in potential human economic development and capital through vocational training, internships, job shadowing, pursuit of a college education and so forth. Overcoming economic hurdles and lack of knowledge regarding how to proceed to reach these goals requires guidance and connection to available resources such as college financial aid assistance, military benefits, accessing vocational rehabilitation services and the like.

As helping professionals, practitioners must realize the importance of employment and the amelioration of poverty in their quest toward healthy living for teens (and/or their families) and young adults in the community. It may be of benefit to bear in mind the significance of Article 23 of the United Nations Declaration of Human Rights. This article clearly states that, "Everyone has the right to work, to free choice of employment, to just and favourable conditions of work and to protection against unemployment" (United Nations, 1948). In addition, it expounds on that point by stating that, "Everyone, without any discrimination, has the right to equal pay for equal work" (United Nations, 1948). Although these articles are not fully implemented in the United States or across the globe, they are admirable aspirations for which to strive. It is vital that mental health practitioners remain vigilant and cognizant of issues such as racial, gender, religious, disability, and sexual orientation discrimination in the lives of our clients. At times, advocacy may pertain to and remain a viable course of action when promoting the health and well-being of our clients and their families.

Adolescence is a time of numerous challenges, one of these being poverty. In fact, in general, more individuals live in poverty in the United States who are under the age of eighteen than in any other age group (McCarter, 2011). In addition, because society is continuing to experience a paradigm shift toward a trained and educated work-force, young adults who are under-trained and under-educated are disadvantaged when seeking gainful employment (Matto, 2011). This in turn, contributes to some young adults earning low wages, and thus, decreased earning power over their lifespan. Encouraging teens and young adults to obtain advanced training or education may benefit them and their future families throughout their entire lives.

Additionally, mental health practitioners and other concerned individuals may advocate for positive change at the community level. For communities to function well and to foster economic success, four forms of community based equity are valuable toward the development of economic growth. These include:

- Jobs that pay fair and above-average wages
- Positions that provide healthcare coverage for employees
- Educational opportunities for community members
- Opportunities for community members to establish good credit ratings (De Vol, 2006, p. 30)

The story "I Can't Find a Job" describes the circumstances of a young adult, who despite staying in school and graduating, cannot find gainful employment in these difficult economic times. Using this story, practitioners could provide emotional support and encouragement to those who find themselves in this discouraging position. Realistic feedback could also be given regarding employment and training opportunities. Connecting clients with any needed community resources such as food, clothing, shelter, and vocational training or college opportunities is also of vital importance.

In the scenario, "Moving," a high-school aged adolescent experiences distress resulting from a parent's job loss. The challenges of having to relocate while in high school because of financial difficulties are explored. Ways to cope with this situation may be built into conversations, stories and drawings involving mental health professionals and those confronting this type of challenging circumstance.

"I Got Fired" describes the scenario of a young adult who is being treated unfairly in the work environment and who is fired from a job that he or she has worked for many years. Emotions of distress and anger are explored. Also, financial stressors and factors dealing with issues of unemployment are examined. This story could be useful when discussing employment, unemployment, discrimination, and work-related behaviors with adolescent and young adult clients. It could serve as a springboard for discussion regarding options and choices regarding employment.

Additional Resources

Chertavian, G. (2012). *A year up: How a pioneering program teaches young adults real skills for real jobs—with real success.* New York: Viking.

Crane, D. R., & Heaton, T. B. (Eds.). (2008). *Handbook of families and poverty.* Thousand Oaks, CA: Sage Publications, Inc.

Neumark, D. (Ed.). (2000). *On the job: Is long-term employment a thing of the past?* New York: Russell Sage Foundation.

Shanks, T. R.W., & Mesmin, D. (2009). Parental expectations and educational outcomes for young African American adults: Do household assets matter? *Race and Social Problems,* 1, 27–35. doi: 10.1007/s12552-009-9001-7.

I Can't Find a Job

They keep on saying that the economy is getting better, but it sure doesn't seem that way to me. I go from place to place asking for work, but it has been months since I graduated and I'm not getting any calls from employers. Did I do something wrong? I just don't get it.

I keep on trying to do everything right. I went to school and graduated just like everyone told me to, but I am still unemployed. I just want a good, full-time position with benefits so I can support myself and save for a place of my own someday. Sometimes I wonder why I even bothered going to school. Maybe I will have to move away from here to try to get a good paying job.

Instructions: Tell, write, or draw the answers to the following questions.

I Can't Find a Job Questions: Level 1

1. How does this young man or woman feel about his or her job search?
2. Do you think he or she will be able to find a good job?
3. What are some positive steps he or she has taken to try to find a job?
4. What are some strengths that he or she could build on to improve his or her chances of getting a good job?
5. How would you finish this story?

I Can't Find a Job Questions: Level 2

1. Has anyone you know ever had a very difficult time finding work?
2. How did he or she feel about not being able to find a job?
3. Did he or she ever find a good job?
4. What helped him or her or could have helped him or her to find a good job?
5. What are some strengths that he or she could have used to improve his or her job search or job skills?
6. What is his or her story?
7. How would you change his or her story if you could?

I Can't Find a Job Questions: Level 3

1. Have you ever had a very difficult time finding a job?
2. How did you feel about this?
3. What are some possible options available to you to help you prepare for your job search?
4. What are some strengths that you could build on to improve your job search skills or work skills?
5. What is your story?
6. How would you change your story if you could?

My Story: Level 4

Instructions: Tell, write, or draw your own story.

Moving

I can't believe we have to move. It's all because my dad lost his stupid job. Now we are leaving right in the middle of my junior year. This is so unfair. I am going to miss everything. All of my friends are here, I'm going to miss going to Prom, and I have to quit my job at the mall. If this had just happened two years from now it wouldn't even matter because I would be in college. I don't understand why he couldn't find something around here.

I don't want to move away from all of my friends. This totally stinks.

Instructions: Tell, write, or draw the answers to the following questions.

Moving Questions: Level 1

1. How does this young man or woman feel about having to move?
2. What are some ways that he or she can cope with moving in a positive manner?
3. How could he or she stay in touch with old friends?
4. What could he or she say or do to adjust to moving to a new school and neighborhood?
5. How would you finish this story?

Moving Questions: Level 2

1. Has anyone you know had to move to a new school or neighborhood?
2. How did he or she cope with the move?
3. How did he or she stay in touch with old friends?
4. What did he or she say or do to adjust to moving to a new school and neighborhood?
5. What is his or her story?
6. How would you change his or her story if you could?

Moving Questions: Level 3

1. Have you ever had to move to a new school or neighborhood?
2. How did you cope with the move?
3. How did you stay in touch with your friends?
4. What did you say or do to adjust to moving to a new school and neighborhood?
5. What is your story?
6. How would you change your story if you could?

My Story: Level 4

Instructions: Tell, write, or draw your own story.

I Got Fired

My boss is such a jerk. So when he told me I was scheduled to work more Saturdays and more nights, when nobody else has to do that, I became very angry. Then, I started thinking about how I haven't gotten a raise in 5 years, when the full-time employees get raises every year, and health benefits. Then I really got mad. So when he told me the next day that I had to come in on Sunday to cover for a full-timer I just couldn't handle it. I stood up for myself and told him that I already had plans that Sunday, and that I just couldn't come in. I told him I didn't feel I was being treated fairly because part-timers didn't get raises or health benefits. And I meant what I said. I am proud of myself for standing up for what I believe in—but unfortunately my supervisor did not feel the same way. He told me that if I felt that way I should go elsewhere. He wished me well, and then he said, "Good luck to you. I am afraid I have to let you go." So basically, I was politely fired after working faithfully at the same job for 5 years. Now what do I do? I don't have a job and I need the money.

Instructions: Tell, write, or draw the answers to the following questions.

I Got Fired Questions: Level 1

1. How does this young man or woman feel about his or her job?
2. How does he or she feel about getting fired?
3. What are some ways that he or she can cope with getting fired?
4. How could he or she have handled this situation differently?
5. How would you finish this story?

I Got Fired Questions: Level 2

1. Has anyone you know had to work at a job where he or she was treated unfairly?
2. Has anyone you know ever been fired from a job?
3. How did he or she cope with getting fired?
4. What is his or her story?
5. How would you change his or her story if you could?

I Got Fired Questions: Level 3

1. Have you ever worked at a job where you were treated unfairly?
2. Have you ever been fired from a job?
3. How did you cope with getting fired?
4. What is your story?
5. How would you change your story if you could?

My Story: Level 4

Instructions: Tell, write, or draw your own story.

Steps I Can Take Activity

Instructions: In each block, write or draw the "steps" or actions you can take to improve your educational and career prospects.

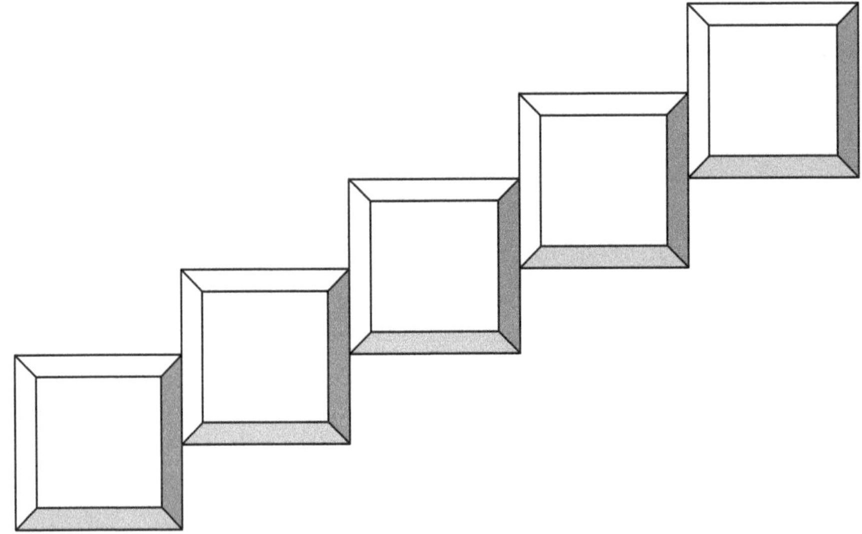

Illness and Disability

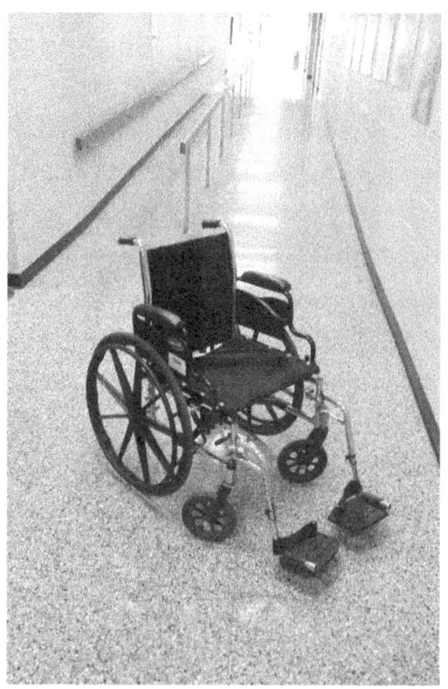

Key Practice Issues and Story Selection

At one point in time, nearly every mental health practitioner will encounter a person in need who is experiencing difficulty adapting to illness or disability of oneself or of a friend or family member. When illness or disability strikes, its ripples tend to be felt by everyone close to the person directly affected, including family, friends, and intimate partners. Depending upon the type, quality, and characteristics of a mental or physical illness or challenge, these ripples may be small or large.

For example, one family's functioning may be temporarily altered by a parent who is unable to work or drive because of injuries sustained in an automobile accident. While yet another family may struggle to adapt and cope with adjusting to the chronic illness of a teenage daughter who requires frequent trips to multiple doctors and expensive medical supplies. In both circumstances, professionals may assist in alleviating stress, promoting development of coping mechanisms, and connecting those in need with special services.

Suggestions for assisting those with illness and disability include:

- Listen to the person in a supportive, caring manner.
- Allow the person to grieve for losses, including loss of physical or mental functioning, loss of income, loss of abilities such as driving, loss of relationships and so forth.
- Connect the individual with resources or agencies that can provide extra assistance with adaptive equipment, medical supplies, and eventually career planning.
- When a practitioner feels a person is ready, gently attempt to guide an individual in discussing and focusing on current abilities and plans for the present and the future. Remember, however, not to minimize the very real grief and loss that the individual has experienced.
- Advocate for the rights of a person on the local, state, and federal levels if human, employment, housing or other civil rights are being violated.

In Tuttle and Tuttle's (1996) book, *Self-esteem and Adjusting with Blindness: The Process of Responding to Life's Demands*, they discuss the process that many individuals experience as they suffer vision loss. This theory may also be applied to others who are adjusting to various disabilities or injuries in their lives. They delineate seven phases of adjustment to blindness including physical or social trauma, shock and denial, mourning and withdrawal, succumbing and depression, reassessment and reaffirmation, coping and mobilization, and self-acceptance and self-esteem. Each person may progress through these stages in a unique manner. In a sense, those who lose their vision move through stages similar to the bereaved, except they are mourning the loss of functioning, both social and physical. This includes adjusting to new methods or techniques of living one's life, and possibly a temporary or permanent change in level of independence. Social and emotional support from practitioners, friends, community and family members is vital during this period of adjustment. It is essential to provide hope for improved quality of life while individuals traverse this precarious terrain while traveling on their journey of adjustment to life with a disability.

During the trauma phase, a person may feel completely overwhelmed with the idea of vision loss. In the shock and denial phase, a teen might feel extreme disbelief that he or she has actually become blind, and may make statements such as "I can't believe this is happening to me." Then, when experiencing mourning and withdrawal, one may emotionally feel badly for oneself and may stop participating in activities that were previously pleasurable. For adolescents or young adults, this may mean that they no longer have the motivation or desire to spend time with friends, boyfriends, or girlfriends.

During the succumbing and depression phase, a person may feel extremely sad or devastated about the vision loss. If this occurs for a prolonged period of time, it may develop into clinical depression. Thorough assessments should be conducted regarding this, and if further psychiatric assessment is needed, referrals and evaluations should be made. Reassessment and reaffirmation will hopefully occur, when individuals make meaning of their experiences and self-reflect. In the coping and mobilization phase, teens and young adults ideally will become more positive in their outlook, and with help from professionals, friends, and family, begin to search for adaptive skills, information, behaviors, and attitudes which will propel them into a brighter future incorporating accommodations for disability into their lives. Hopefully, many clients will progress to the final phase of self-acceptance and self-esteem. This is when individuals have accepted vision loss or blindness as a part of their lives, realizing that they still can live fulfilling and successful lives (Tuttle & Tuttle, 1996).

Conceptually, even after individuals' have adjusted to living as persons with disabilities, they may still encounter misunderstanding and discrimination in their personal, academic, and professional lives. One suggestion for assisting those confronting disability discrimination is by approaching the issue from a blended perspective of utilizing various theories applicable in disability oriented practice. Components of building on clients strengths, encouraging empowerment, promoting resiliency, developing environments inclusive of differing abilities, encouraging appropriate medical care, and advocating to end discrimination based on disability all comprise elements important to positive practice involving those with disabilities (Raske, 2005).

In the vignette, "The Accident," a young person experiences a traumatic accident in which he or she is severely injured. The young adult feels depressed regarding the loss of physical functioning resulting from the accident. Not only can he or she no longer walk, but the character is upset because he or she had been a basketball player previously, and is mourning the loss of playing the game, status, and team affiliation. Supportive counseling is crucial during this difficult period of loss and adjustment. When ready, plans for the future may be incorporated into therapeutic storytelling surrounding issues of adjustment.

The story, "My Arthritis," addresses the various issues an adolescent encounters when living with a chronic condition that sometimes limits his or her activities of daily living. Due to the variable nature of this illness, friends and family sometimes ignore or lack the knowledge and insight needed to support this person to overcome challenges. In addition, the individual is confronted with stressors of medication management, multiple physician visits, and weight gain associated with medication, that peers and others may not experience. Supportive counseling, active listening, and restorying both challenges and strengths with a skilled clinician may assist in building coping skills of someone identifying with this character.

In "Being Blind," a young person experiences feelings of grief, loss, and anger surrounding issues of severe vision loss. Individuals may relate to this experience if they have lost their sight or if they have become severely disabled in another way. These feelings of grief and anger can occur when someone has become severely disabled. However, these may be overcome with supportive counseling and new or modified goals for the future, based on each person's desires, abilities, and accommodations.

Additional Resources

Kennedy, A., Sloman, F., Douglass, J. A., & Sawyer, S. M. (2007). Young people with chronic illness: The approach to transition. *Internal Medicine Journal*, 37, 555–560. DOI: 10:1111/j.1445-5994.2007.01440.x

May, G. E., & Raske, M. B. (Eds.). (2005). *Ending disability discrimination: Strategies for social workers.* Boston, MA: Pearson Education, Inc.

Silverstone, B., Lang, M. A., Rosenthal, B., & Faye, E. E. (2000). *The Lighthouse handbook on vision impairment and vision rehabilitation.* New York: Oxford University Press/Lighthouse International.

Slivinske, J. (2013). The job club support group: Multiple disabilities. In L. M. Grobman & J. Clements (Eds.), *Riding the mutual aid bus and other adventures in group work: A days in the lives of social workers collection* (pp. 87–93). Harrisburg, PA: White Hat Communications.

Tuttle, D., & Tuttle, N. (1996). *Self-esteem and adjusting with blindness: The process of responding to life's demands.* Springfield, IL: Charles C. Thomas.

The Accident

Ever since the accident, I've had to use a wheelchair. They say I might have to be in it forever. I don't really know what to think about all of this. I used to be so athletic, and was a standout player on the basketball team. Now I can't even walk! I mean really, that's pretty unfair. They say that as I'm further into my recovery, that I might be able to play wheelchair basketball. I don't really want to, but what choice do I have? I suppose that this is part of my life now.

Instructions: Tell, write, or draw the answers to the following questions.

The Accident Questions: Level 1

1. How does this young man or woman feel about his or her severe injury?
2. Do this person's friends and family understand what he or she is going through?
3. What are some healthy ways that he or she can cope with the injury?
4. What are some strengths that he or she could build on to enhance his or her coping skills?
5. How would you finish this story?

The Accident Questions: Level 2

1. Has anyone you know experienced a severe injury?
2. How does this make him or her feel?
3. Do this person's friends and family understand what he or she is going through?
4. What are some healthy ways that he or she can cope with having a severe injury?
5. What are some strengths that he or she could build on to enhance his or her coping skills?
6. How would you finish this story?

The Accident Questions: Level 3

1. Have you ever experienced a severe injury?
2. How do feel about your injury?
3. Do your friends and family understand what you are going through?
4. What are some possible ways you can cope with your injury?
5. What are some strengths that you could build on to improve your coping skills?
6. What is your story?
7. How would you change your story if you could?

My Story: Level 4

Instructions: Tell, write, or draw your own story.

My Arthritis

Sometimes my friends don't really understand what I'm going through. I'm only sixteen, but I have arthritis. They think that only old people get arthritis, but that's simply not true. I know—because I have it and it stinks. Sometimes I feel really good, but sometimes I feel really bad, and I never can predict how I am really going to feel.

When I have an arthritis flare up, I feel exhausted and I hurt all over. I really ache, and I'm not supposed to do a lot when that happens. I have to limit my activities and take it easy. When I feel well though, I can do just about anything, if I don't overdo it. Sometimes people think I am faking feeling sick, but I am definitely not faking!

I also have to take all of this stupid medicine! I take about 10 pills a day and have to get shots sometimes to control the flares. It is a real pain to take the medicine and it makes me more likely to catch an infection—so I can't even be around a person who has a cold because I could become extremely sick. Some of the medicine makes me gain weight, so I have to constantly watch my diet. I am tired of visiting the doctor all of the time too. I wish this stupid arthritis would just go away!

Instructions: Tell, write, or draw the answers to the following questions.

My Arthritis Questions: Level 1

1. How does this young man or woman feel about having arthritis?
2. Do this person's friends and family understand what he or she is going through?
3. What are some ways that he or she can educate friends and family about arthritis?
4. What are some healthy ways that he or she can cope with having arthritis?
5. What are some strengths that he or she could build on to enhance his or her coping skills?
6. How would you finish this story?

My Arthritis Questions: Level 2

1. Does anyone you know have arthritis or another chronic illness?
2. How does this make him or her feel?
3. Do this person's friends and family understand what he or she is going through?
4. What are some ways that he or she can educate friends and family about arthritis or another illness?
5. What are some healthy ways that he or she can cope with having a chronic condition?
6. What are some strengths that he or she could build on to enhance his or her coping skills?
7. How would you finish this story?

My Arthritis Questions: Level 3

1. Do you have arthritis or another chronic illness?
2. How do feel about having your illness?
3. Do your friends and family understand what you are going through?

4. What are some possible ways you can cope with your chronic condition?
5. What are some strengths that you could build on to improve your coping skills?
6. What is your story?
7. How would you change your story if you could?

My Story: Level 4

Instructions: Tell, write, or draw your own story.

Being Blind

Sometimes I wish I was just like everyone else. I wish I could just do all of the things I used to be able to do, like drive a car or watch a movie. Now I have to rely on everyone to take me everywhere. I can't stand it that my parents have to drive me over to my girlfriend's house, to the store, and everywhere else I even want to go. They treat me like I am a child. I hate being blind. There's just so much I feel like I can't do anymore, even though I still want to so desperately. If it weren't for my stupid genetics, I'd still be able to see. I would give anything to be able to see again . . .

I used to be just like you. I didn't know how good I had it and how easy my life was. I could drive, read, and see how pretty my girlfriend is. Now those are all just memories. I'll never see again... I really hate my life right now. I don't know how I am going to be able to survive all of this.

Instructions: Text, write, or draw the answers to the following questions.

Being Blind Questions: Level 1

1. How does this young man feel about losing his sight?
2. Do this person's friends and family understand what he is going through?
3. What are some ways that he can educate friends and family about what it is like to be blind?
4. What are some healthy ways that he can cope with all of the grief and losses that he has experienced because of his loss of vision?
5. What are some strengths that he could build on to enhance his coping skills?
6. How would you finish this story?

Being Blind Questions: Level 2

1. Is anyone you know blind or visually impaired?
2. How does this make him or her feel?
3. Do this person's friends and family understand what he or she is going through?
4. What are some ways that he or she can educate friends and family about blindness and visual impairments?
5. What are some healthy ways that he or she can cope with blindness or vision loss?
6. What are some strengths that he or she could build on to enhance his or her coping skills?
7. How would you finish this story?

Being Blind Questions: Level 3

1. Are you blind or visually impaired?
2. How do feel about your blindness or visual impairment?
3. Do your friends and family understand what you are going through?
4. What are some possible ways you can cope with the losses you have experienced as a result of your blindness or visual impairment?

5. What are some strengths that you could build on to improve your coping skills?
6. What is your story?
7. How would you change your story if you could?

My Story: Level 4

Instructions: Tell, write, or draw your own story.

Steps I Can Take Activity

Instructions: In each segment of the circle, tell, write, or draw your own perceptions of your losses, abilities, things you are not sure about and areas in which you can grow.

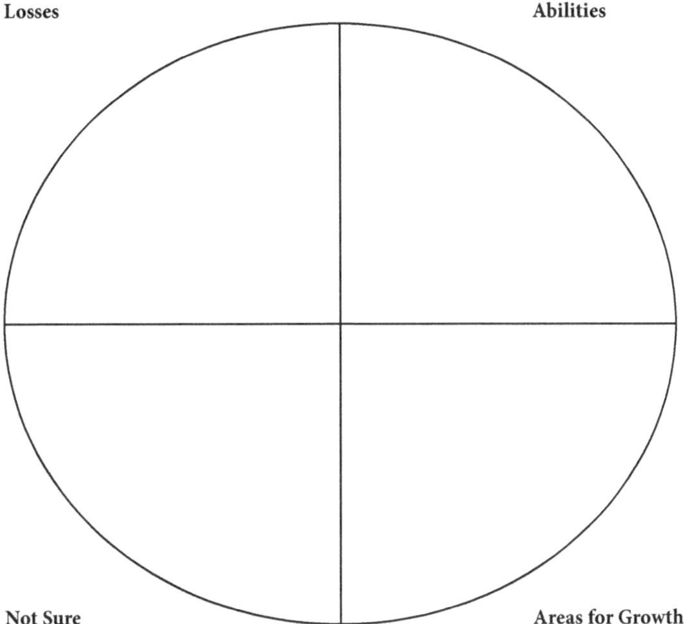

24

School Issues

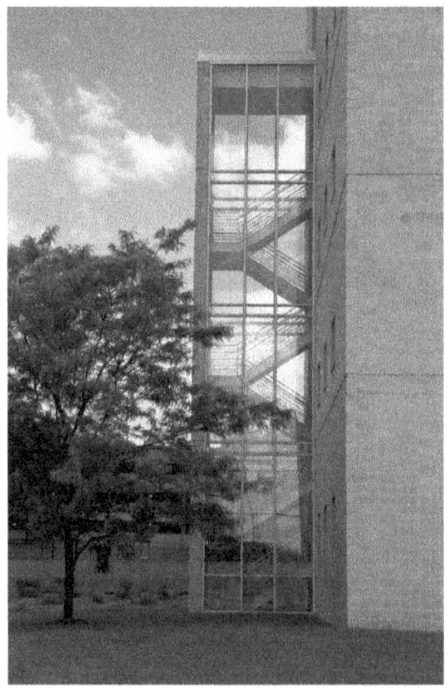

Key Practice Issues and Story Selection

Most individuals of high school and young adult ages have encountered some type of difficulty with school issues, both positive and negative. These challenges encompass anything along the continuum from extreme academic success to academic suspension or failure. Many, if not the majority, of social interactions and relationships occur within the context of the school environment for adolescents of high school and college age.

Stress and anxiety regarding earning high marks, test-taking, or low grades and failure, may contribute to feelings of academic pressure and tension. Students may benefit from exercises and activities such as the stories presented in this book in order to learn methods, techniques, and interventions that delineate teachable skills. Modeling and role playing how to cope with these particular stressors may also be of benefit.

For college-age students, test-taking may provoke an anxiety related experience, bringing to mind feelings of panic, stress, and fear of failure. Some experience test-anxiety, which manifests itself in altered cognition and physiological responses in the testing environment. These students may need assistance to remain calm and focused in the testing or evaluative situation (Cizek & Burg, 2006). Positive interactions with one's professors during office hours may help to alleviate this anxiety and allow for increased understanding of any unclear or challenging material. Campus support services such as tutoring, peer mentoring, and study groups may additionally benefit certain students in need of supplemental services, encouragement, and assistance. For students with poor study habits, review courses surrounding the particulars of how to study and methods to improve organization and efficiency may be valuable.

For those students predisposed to naturally occurring high anxiety, meditation, breathing exercises, and relaxation exercises may be practiced with the client in-session. These rehearsals may then be applied in the real test-taking environment. Also, those with a certified disability may be eligible for special accommodations through the university's office of disability services. Some of these possible accommodations for a student with an anxiety disorder, or other disabling physical or mental impairment include: extended time to take exams, a quiet location to take exams, a reader to read the exam aloud, a scribe, use of a computer to take an exam allowing for the use of spell-check, and similar adaptations. Many other special accommodations may be provided based on the specific needs and limitations of a person with a physical or mental challenge.

Many techniques may provide a decline in the level of anxiety felt by students experiencing emotional distress regarding academic pressure or test-related anxiety. These include the following methods for management of anxiety (Stallard, 2009) and can be applied to those with school-related anxiety concerns:

- Controlled breathing may be practiced before, during, and after taking examinations. This technique may be modified to suit the preferences and needs of individuals, and it basically involves slowly breathing deeply, holding the breath, and then slowly releasing the breath. Thinking soothing words or phrases such as "mellow" or "I am relaxed" may provide additional comfort to some people.
- Exercise or physical activities, may provide relief from anxiety and may be timed to coordinate with planned stressors, such as exams or the writing of final term papers, to optimize stress reduction.
- Using mental challenges to distract oneself from his or her own thoughts may help some teens and young adults to better cope with anxiety. Examples of simple mental challenges include naming everyone a person knows whose name begins with the letter M, or counting backward from 100 by 2s.

- Another technique involving distraction for pre-exam anxiety involves focusing one's attention on details in the immediate surroundings. The person may then think about all of the details or speak them aloud, depending on the circumstances. For example, the person may internally or aloud say "The room is bright yellow; it smells like flowery perfume; the windows are clean; and the floor tile is square with black, green and yellow squiggly lines." This focus on external stimuli in the environment redirects attention away from anxiety-provoking thoughts within one's mind.
- Progressive muscle relaxation involves systematically tightening and then relaxing various muscle groups, and may provide relief from stress or anxiety. This may be conducted prior to test-taking, or inconspicuously during the time of the exam.
- Guided imagery may assist some teens and young adults prior to examinations. They may choose a relaxing or comforting setting to imagine in their minds. It may be an amusement park on a sunny day, a calm and serene lake, the ocean, or any place that provides feelings of positive emotional responses. The individual then envisions that particular environment, including imagining sensory experiences of how the place looks, smells, and sounds.
- When studying, it is sometimes desirable to take time-out breaks to relax and engage in some calming activities to rejuvenate one's mind. These activities will vary from person-to-person, but may include texting a friend, listening to music, playing a video game, or talking with a family member. Encourage teens and young adults to find what activities they find pleasurable and relaxing. The activities that they discover now may provide fun, relaxation, and anxiety relief throughout their lives.

The stories "The Pressure" and "Finals" address the concerns students may face regarding academic success and anxiety surrounding test-taking. These stories may benefit students who may readily relate to current academic stressors. Both vignettes may serve as springboards for discussions and present opportunities for artistic interventions and expression. In addition, individuals may be taught relaxation techniques and methods.

In "I Hate School," a young person is concerned and worried about negative school performance and possible academic failure. He or she is anxious regarding how this will affect his or her future. In addition, apprehension abounds surrounding issues involving how academic troubles will impact this person's relationship with his or her parents and others. When practicing with a person who relates to this scenario, linking with and implementing both academic and social supports may be beneficial. Short-term and long-term planning may assist in solidifying a clearer, productive path for a young person's future.

Additional Resources

Cizek, G. J., & Burg, S. S. (2006). *Addressing test anxiety in a high-stakes environment: Strategies for classrooms and schools.* Thousand Oaks, CA: Corwin Press.

Franklin, C., Harris, M. B., & Allen-Meares, P. (Eds.). (2006). *The school services sourcebook: A guide for school-based professionals.* New York: Oxford University Press.

Johnson, S. (2000). *Taking the anxiety out of taking tests: A step—by—step guide.* New York: Barnes & Noble Books.

Winslade, J. M., & Monk, G. D. (2007). *Narrative counseling in schools: Powerful and brief* (2nd ed.). Thousand Oaks, CA: Corwin Press.

The Pressure

I'm doing really well in school and getting excellent grades—but sometimes I just feel like I can't take the pressure. My parents say that the better I do now and the harder the courses are that I take, the more of a chance I will have of gaining entrance to an outstanding university. I know that they are right. I'm also volunteering at a local nursing home and an animal shelter which I really enjoy, but doing these types of community service will hopefully help me to earn scholarships as well.

It just feels overwhelming sometimes though—like it is just too much to handle. I am afraid to even get a B on my report card because it might affect my chance of winning a scholarship or getting accepted at an outstanding school. I just want to be good enough... Sometimes before exams I get extremely nervous and start to sweat. I just wish I could relax a little bit more about everything.

Instructions: Tell, write, or draw the answers to the following questions.

The Pressure Questions: Level 1

1. How does this young man or woman feel about earning high marks in school?
2. What are the expectations of his or her family regarding attending a university?
3. What are some ways that he or she can cope with this pressure in a positive manner?
4. What are some strengths that he or she could build on to enhance his or her coping skills?
5. How would you finish this story?

The Pressure Questions: Level 2

1. Does anyone you know experience this kind of pressure and anxiety regarding school?
2. What are the expectations of his or her parents regarding school?
3. How does this make him or her feel?
4. What are some possible ways he or she can cope with school pressure and anxiety?
5. What are some strengths that he or she could build on to improve his or her coping ability?
6. What is his or her story?
7. How would you change his or her story if you could?

The Pressure Questions: Level 3

1. Do you ever feel pressure or anxiety regarding school?
2. How do your parents feel about your school performance?
3. How does this make you feel?
4. What are some possible ways you can cope with school pressure and anxiety?
5. What are some strengths that you could build on to improve your coping skills?
6. What is your story?
7. How would you change your story if you could?

My Story: Level 4

Instructions: Tell, write, or draw your own story.

Finals

I absolutely hate finals week. I get so nervous that I feel like I am going to explode. I usually end up doing alright on the exams, but I can't stand how stressed out and anxious I am the entire week. Sometimes, when I sit down to take the test, I break out in a sweat, and my mind goes totally blank! My heart starts racing and I can feel it pounding inside of my chest. And this is after I have studied for days to master the material, and I actually know and understand the material.

I wish I could find a way to relax more—or just never take a final exam again!

Instructions: Tell, write, or draw the answers to the following questions.

Finals Questions: Level 1

1. How does this young man or woman feel about taking tests in school?
2. What are some ways that he or she can cope with test-anxiety in a positive manner?
3. What are some strengths that he or she could build on to enhance his or her coping skills?
4. How would you finish this story?

Finals Questions: Level 2

1. Does anyone you know experience this kind of test-anxiety?
2. How does this make him or her feel?
3. What are some possible ways he or she can cope with test-anxiety?
4. What are some strengths that he or she could build on to improve his or her coping ability?
5. What is his or her story?
6. How would you change his or her story if you could?

Finals Questions: Level 3

1. Do you ever feel pressure or anxiety regarding tests?
2. How does this make you feel?
3. What are some possible ways you can cope with test-anxiety?
4. What are some strengths that you could build on to improve your coping skills?
5. What is your story?
6. How would you change your story if you could?

My Story: Level 4

Instructions: Tell, write, or draw your own story.

I Hate School

I hate school. I don't know why I even bother going to school. I have never done that well in it, and now I am close to flunking out. I am on academic probation, and I don't even know how I am going to bring my grades up. I am tired of trying, and it just seems like nothing is going right for me.

My parents are worried about me, but my mom never graduated, so I don't see how she can talk. I guess she wants a better life for me than what she has. I really want to make her happy and I really want to graduate, but I just don't know how I'm ever going to be able to do that.

Instructions: Tell, write, or draw the answers to the following questions.

I Hate School Questions: Level 1

1. How does this young man or woman feel about being on academic probation?
2. What are the expectations of his or her family regarding school performance?
3. What are some ways that he or she can cope with these academic challenges in a positive manner?
4. What are some strengths that he or she could build on to enhance his or her coping skills?
5. How would you finish this story?

I Hate School Questions: Level 2

1. Has anyone you know ever experienced this kind of stress and anxiety because of poor grades in school?
2. What were the expectations of his or her parents regarding school performance?
3. How did all of this academic stress make him or her feel?
4. What are some ways he or she coped with academic stress?
5. What are some strengths that he or she built on to improve his or her coping ability?
6. What is his or her story?
7. How would you change his or her story if you could?

I Hate School Questions: Level 3

1. Do you ever feel stress or anxiety regarding school performance?
2. How do your parents feel about your school performance?
3. How does this make you feel?
4. What are some possible ways you can cope with these academic challenges?
5. What are some strengths that you could build on to improve your coping skills?
6. What is your story?
7. How would you change your story if you could?

My Story: Level 4

Instructions: Tell, write, or draw your own story.

Relaxation Exercise

Instructions: In your mind, go to a place or a time that makes you feel at peace and relaxed. Examples may include when you are sitting by a lake, having fun with friends, or eating a comforting food. Practice this technique now with your therapist, friend or family member. You may also use this technique before an exam or another stressful life event. If you like, write or draw about your place or time that makes you feel peaceful and relaxed.

Imagined Traits Relaxation Activity

Instructions: Imagine how someone who is confident and relaxed would handle taking an exam or face a difficult situation. Pretend you have the qualities and skills of stress management that this person possesses. Practice using those skills in an imaginary scenario with a friend, family member, or therapist.

25

General Activities for All Practice Areas

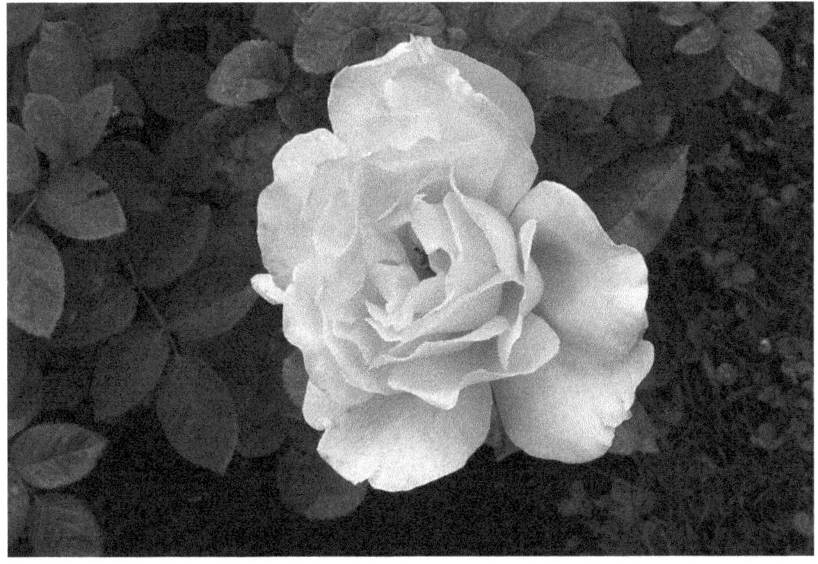

Key Practice Issues and Story Selection

The following activities may be used to assist clients with a wide variety of challenges and strengths. The activities are designed to be general, and are applicable for many areas of practice. They may be personalized at the discretion of the clinician, in order to meet specific client needs.

Where Am I? Activity

Instructions: In the center circle, write or draw where you would like to be in the future. In the outer circles, write or draw what you need to do to get to where you would like to be in the future.

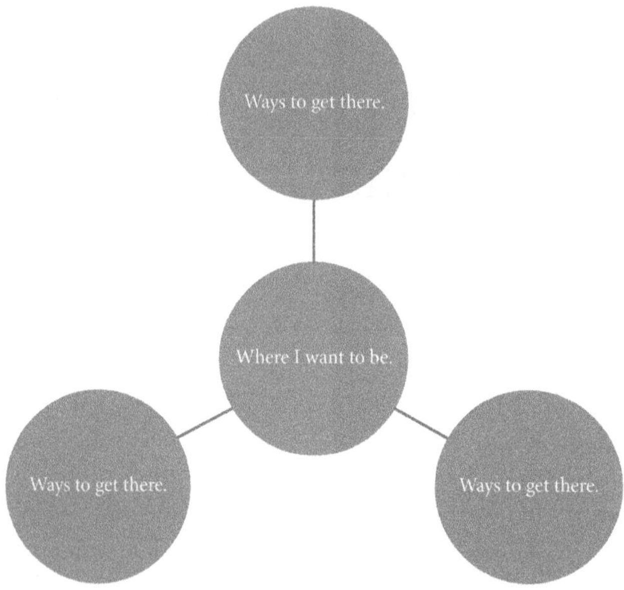

Relaxation Exercise Activity

Instructions: In your mind, go to a place or a time that makes you feel at peace and relaxed. Examples may include when you are sitting by a lake, having fun with friends, or eating a comforting food. Practice this technique now with your therapist, friend or family member. You may also use this technique before an exam or another stressful life event. If you like, write or draw about your place or time that makes you feel peaceful and relaxed.

Imagined Traits Relaxation Activity

Instructions: Imagine how someone who is confident and relaxed would handle taking an exam or face a difficult situation. Pretend you have the qualities and skills of stress management that this person possesses. Practice using those skills in an imaginary scenario with a friend, family member, or therapist.

My Story

Instructions: Tell, write, or draw your own story about your life.

Strengths Activity: The PLAN Method of Intervention

Instructions: Tell, write, or draw the answers to the following questions or statements.

Positive action creates positive lifestyles

What are some positive actions you can take in your life?

Look to the future

What do you want to accomplish in the future?

Activate your strengths, inside and out

What are some of your strengths?

Never give up on yourself

When I feel like quitting or giving up I will . . .

Activity: Positive Action Creates Positive Change

Instructions: In the diagram below, write or draw the actions you can take to improve your life.

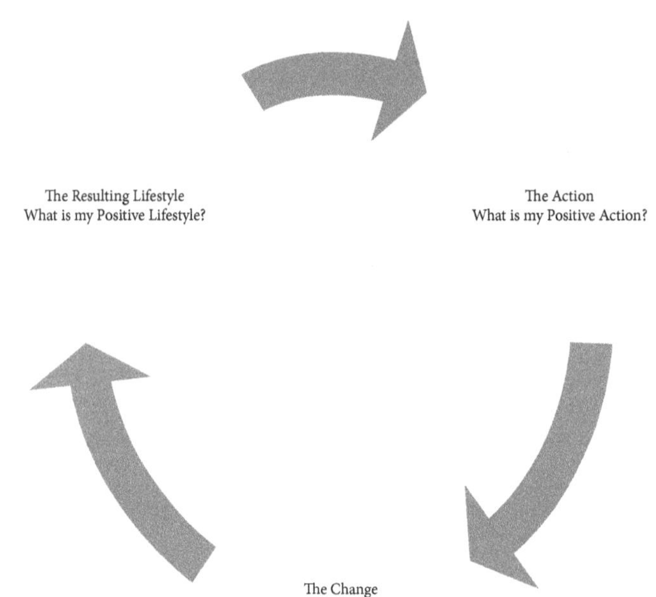

Strengths Activity: Look to the Future

Instructions: Tell, write, or draw the answers to the following statements to help you to look toward the future. With the help of your friend, parent, or therapist, make a plan to accomplish your goals. Set the plan into action, if you desire.

Tomorrow I would like to . . .
One week from now I would like to . . .
One month from now I would like to . . .
Six months from now I would like to . . .
One year from now I would like to . . .
Two years from now I would like to . . .
Five years from now I would like to . . .
Ten years from now I would like to . . .
Twenty years from now I would like to . . .

Strengths Activity: My Plan Leads to My Future

Instructions: Based upon the previous activity "Look to the Future," choose a time period and set goals to work toward your plans for the future. Tell, write, or draw how you plan to work toward your goals.

Example:

Goal ⇨ Two years from now, I would like to attend college. My goal to work toward this is to research five different colleges on the Internet, and to figure out how I need to apply for school and how to apply for financial aid.

Goal ⇨

Goal ⇨

Writing Activity

Instructions: Free write about the following. There is no right or wrong answer.

Who am I?

Who am I becoming?

Thinking Outside the Box about Yourself

Instructions: Write or draw, outside of the box provided, as many unique, quirky, fun and positive qualities about yourself as you can.

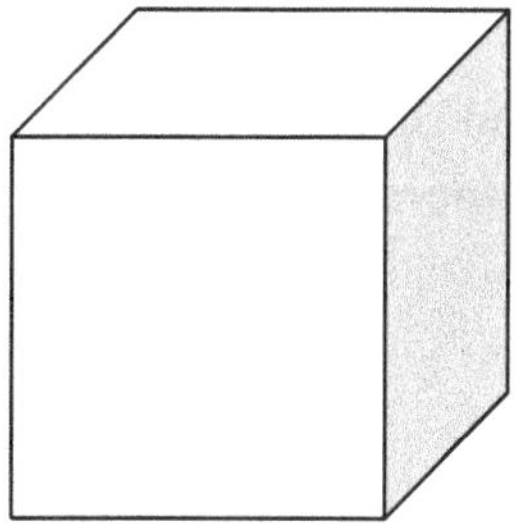

Strengths and Areas Needing Growth in Your Community Activity

Instructions: Tell, write, or draw the answers to the following questions.

1. What are some positive aspects of your community?
2. What activities would you like to participate in or organizations would you like to join in your community? (e.g. health clubs, gyms, social organizations, religious groups, and so forth)
3. What aspects of your community need to be improved?
4. How could someone or an organization begin to move toward positive change in your community?

Create a Video Game Activity

Instructions: Create the plot and characters for a video game that you would like to be a character in. You may be yourself or have another character stand for you. Be creative and have fun!

Steps I Can Take Activity

Instructions: In each block, write or draw the "steps" or actions you can take to improve your educational and career prospects.

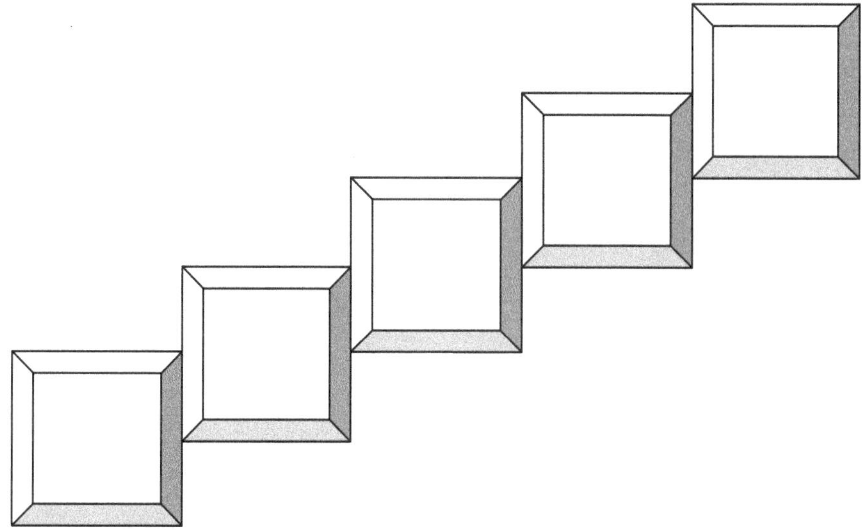

What Are My Options?

Instructions: Tell, write, or draw the answers to the following questions.

Is attending college an option?
Is taking a training course an option?
Is getting a better job an option?
Is getting an apartment with or without a roommate an option?
Is moving to a new city or state an option?

Poem Activity

Instructions: Write a poem about what is happening in your life.

Steps I Can Take Activity

Instructions: In each segment of the circle, write or draw your own perceptions of your losses, abilities, things you are not sure about and areas in which you can grow.

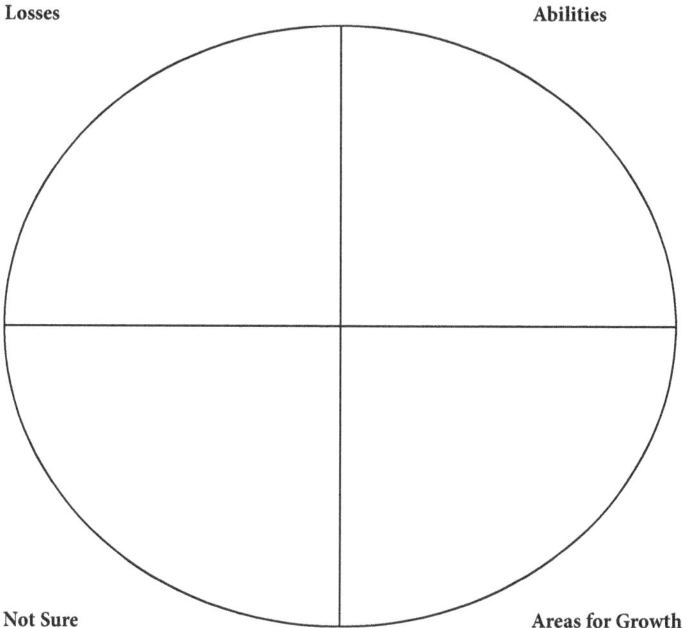

My Sexuality Activity

Instructions: Tell, write, or draw the answers to the following questions.

1. What are your values and beliefs about sexuality and becoming sexually active with someone?
2. How long do you feel you should know someone before becoming sexually active?
3. Should you be married before becoming sexually active?
4. Do you feel you are emotionally prepared enough and mature enough to become sexually active with a particular person?
5. What are some possible positive and negative consequences of becoming sexually active?

Personal Choices Activity

Instructions: Tell, write, or draw the answers to the following statements and questions.

1. Tell, write, or draw any positive things about birth control that you can think of.
2. Tell, write, or draw any negative things about birth control that you can think of.
3. Will you or do you choose to use birth control? Why or why not?

Coping Skills Activity

Write or draw four activities you can participate in to help you to cope positively.

Write or draw two people who you can spend time with or talk with to help you cope.

Write or draw four ways that are not helping you to cope.

Lifemap Activity

Instructions: Write or draw the story of your life.

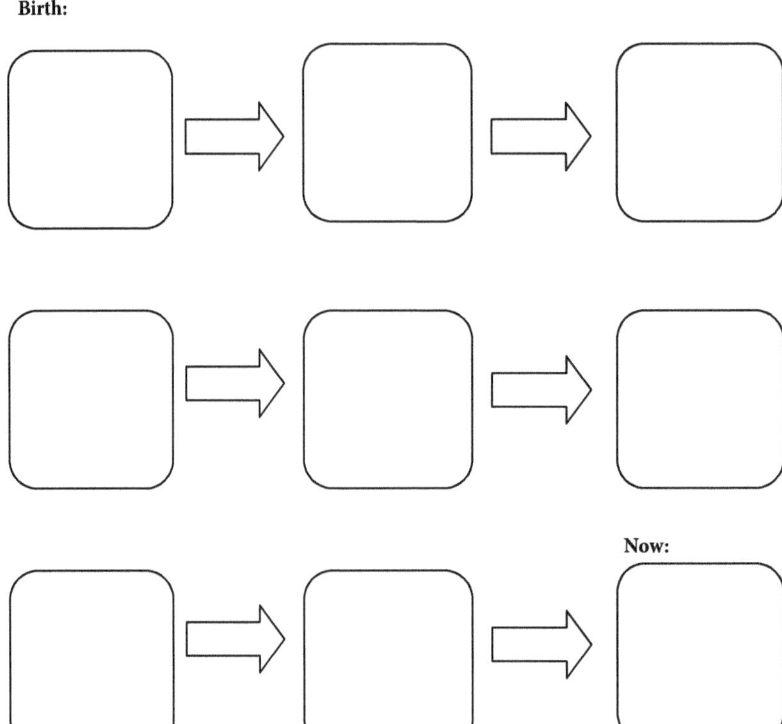

References

American Psychiatric Association. (2000). *Diagnostic and statistical manual of mental disorders* (4th ed., Text Revision). Washington, DC: Author.

Ashford, J. B., & LeCroy, C. W. (2010). *Human behavior in the social environment: A multidimensional perspective* (4th ed.). Belmont, CA: Wadsworth.

Besa, D. (1994). Evaluating narrative family therapy using single system research designs. *Research on Social Work Practice,* 4, 309–326.

Blundell, S. (2001). Psychotherapy with bereaved adolescents. In G. Baruch (Ed.), *Community-based psychotherapy with young people: Evidence and innovation in practice* (pp. 103–114). East Sussex, UK: Brunner-Routledge.

Brown, S. A., McGue, M., Maggs, J., Schulenberg, J., Hingson, R., Swartzwelder, S., et al. (2008). A developmental perspective on alcohol and youths 16 to 20 years of age. *Pediatrics,* 121(Suppl 4), S290–S310.

Carrell, S. (2000). *Group exercises for adolescents: A manual for therapists* (2nd ed). Thousand Oaks, CA: Sage Publications, Inc.

Cashin, A. (2008). Narrative therapy: A psychotherapeutic approach in the treatment of adolescents with Asperger's Disorder. *Journal of Child and Adolescent Psychiatric Nursing,* 21(1), 48–56.

Centers for Disease Control, National Center of Health Statistics. (2006). *Public use data file and documentation: Multiple cause of death for ICD-10 2003 data.* (book on CD-ROM). Hyattsville, MD. National Center of Health Statistics.

Centers for Disease Control and Prevention. (2008). *Sexual violence: Facts at a glance.* Retrieved June 15, 2011, from http://www.cdc.gov/ViolencePrevention/sexualviolence/datasources.html.

Chartier, K. G., Hesselbrock, M. N., & Hesselbrock, V. M. (2011). Alcohol problems in young adults transitioning from adolescence to adulthood: The association with race and gender. *Addictive Behaviors,* 36, 167–174. doi: 10.1016/j.addbeh.2010.10.007

Chen, C. S., & Farruggia, S. (2002). Culture and adolescent development. *Online Readings in Psychology and Culture,* 6(1), 1–12. dx.doi.org/10.9707/2307-0919, 1113.

Cizek, G. J., & Burg, S. S. (2006). *Addressing test anxiety in a high-stakes environment: Strategies for classrooms and schools.* Thousand Oaks, CA: Corwin Press.

Clark-Stewart, A. & Dunn, J. (2006). *Families count: Effects on child and adolescent development.* New York: Cambridge University Press.

Coleman, V. D., & Farris-Dufrene, P. M. (1996). *Art therapy & psychotherapy: Blending two therapeutic approaches.* Washington, DC: Accelerated Development/Taylor & Francis Group.

Connor, D. F. (2002). *Aggression and antisocial behavior in children and adolescents: Research and treatment.* New York: Guilford Press.

Coulehan, R., Friedlander, M., & Heatherington, L. (1998). Transforming narratives: A change event in constructivist family therapy. *Family Process,* 37, 17–33.

Crawford, R., Brown, B., & Crawford, P. (2004). *Storytelling in therapy.* Cheltenham, UK: Nelson Thornes Ltd.

Degges-White, S. (2011). Introduction to the use of expressive arts in counseling. In S. Degges-White & N. L. Davis (Eds.), *Integrating the expressive arts into counseling practice: Theory-based interventions* (pp. 1–6). New York: Springer Publishing Company.

DeLucia-Waack, J. L. (2006). *Leading psychoeducational groups for children and adolescents*. Thousand Oaks, CA: Sage.

De Vol, P. E. (2006). *Facilitator notes for getting ahead in a just-gettin'- by world: Building your resources for a better life*. Highlands, TX: Aha! Process, Inc.

Dishion, T. J., Kavanagh, K., Schneiger, A., Nelson, S., & Kaufman, N. (2002). Preventing early adolescent substance use: A family-centered strategy for public middle school. In R. L. Spoth, K. Kavanagh, & T. J. Dishion (Eds.), Universal family-centered prevention strategies: Current findings and critical issues for public health impact [Special issue]. *Prevention Science*, 3, 191–201.

Divinyi, J. E. (1995). Storytelling: An enjoyable and effective therapeutic tool. *Contemporary Family Therapy*, 17(1), 27–37.

Erford, B. T., Eaves, S. H., Bryant, E. M., & Young, K. A. (2010). 35 *techniques every counselor should know*. Upper Saddle River, NJ: Merrill/Pearson Education, Inc.

Etchison, M., & Kleist, D. M. (2000). Review of narrative therapy: Research and utility. *The Family Journal: Counseling and Therapy for Couples and Families*, 8(1), 61–66.

Ferro, A. (2006). *Psychoanalysis as therapy and storytelling*. London, UK: Routledge.

Field, T., Diego, M. & Sanders, C. (2002). Adolescents' parent and peer relationships. *Adolescence*, 37, 121–130.

Fraley, R. C., & Davis, K. E. (1997). Attachment formation and transfer in young adults' close friendships and romantic relationships. *Personal Relationships*, 4: 131–144. doi: 10.1111/j.1475-6811.1997.tb00135.x

Gabel, K., & Johnston, D. (1995). *Children of incarcerated parents*. New York: Lexington Books.

Gardner, R. A. (1970). The mutual storytelling technique: Use in the treatment of a child with post-traumatic neurosis. *American Journal of Psychotherapy*, 24, 419–439.

Gardner, R. A. (1971). *Therapeutic communication with children: The mutual storytelling technique*. New York: Science House.

Gardner, R. A. (1972). The mutual storytelling technique in the treatment of anger inhibition problems. *International Journal of Child Psychotherapy*, 1(1), 34–64.

Gardner, R. A. (1974). The mutual storytelling technique in the treatment of psychogenic problems secondary to minimal brain dysfunction. *Journal of Learning Disabilities*, 7(3), 14–22.

Gurian, M. (2002). *The wonder of girls: Understanding the hidden nature of our daughters*. New York: Atria Books.

Hair, E. C., Moore, K. A., Garrett, S. B., Ling, T., & Cleveland, K. (2008). The continued importance of quality parent-adolescent relationships during late adolescence. *Journal of Research on Adolescence*, 18(1), 187–200.

Harvey, J. H., & Fine, M. A. (2010). *Children of divorce: Stories of loss and growth*. New York: Routledge.

Hickman, L. J., Jaycox, L. H., & Aronoff, J. (2004). Dating violence among adolescents: Prevalence, gender distribution, and prevention program effectiveness. *Trauma, Violence, & Abuse*, 5(2), 123–142.

Hyde, J. S., & DeLamater, J. D. (2006). *Understanding human sexuality* (9th ed). New York: McGraw Hill Higher Education.

Johnson, L. C., & Yanca, S. J. (2004). *Social work practice: A generalist approach* (8th ed). Boston, MA: Pearson Education.

Kirst-Ashman, K. K. (2011). *Human behavior in the macro social environment: An empowerment approach to understanding communities, organizations, and groups* (3rd ed). Belmont, CA: Brooks/Cole, Cengage Learning.

Kübler-Ross, E. (1969). *On death and dying*. New York: Macmillan.

Leone, D. (2011). Leading causes of brain injuries in children. *Inside Children's: A Publication of Akron Children's Hospital, Spring*, 3.

Lerner, R. M., Jacobs, F. & Wertlieb, D. (2003). *Handbook of applied developmental science, Vol.* 1. Thousand Oaks, CA: Sage Publications.

Levine, L. E., & Munsch, J. (2011). *Child development: An active learning approach*. Thousand Oaks, CA: Sage Publications, Inc.

Lewis, V. E. (2007). The woman who wanted to lie on the floor: A social constructionist use of metaphor in a tale of two clients. In G. W. Burns (Ed.), *Healing with stories: Your casebook collection for using therapeutic metaphors* (pp. 79–99). Hoboken, NJ: John Wiley & Sons, Inc.

Ma, C. Q., & Huebner, E. S. (2008). Attachment relationships and adolescents' life satisfaction: Some relationships matter more to girls than boys. *Psychology in the Schools*, 45, 177–190. doi: 10.1002/pits.20288

Malchiodi, C. A. (2003). Preface. In C. A. Malchiodi (Ed.), *Handbook of art therapy* (pp. ix–iii). New York: The Guilford Press.

Mannion, M. P. (2011). Existential theory. In S. Degges-White & N. L. Davis (Eds.), *Integrating the expressive arts into counseling practice: Theory-based interventions* (pp. 87–100). New York: Springer Publishing Company.

Matsakis, A. (2003). *The rape recovery handbook*. San Francisco, CA: New Harbinger.

Matto, H. C. (2003). Young adulthood. In E. D. Hutchison (Ed.), *Dimensions of human behavior: The changing life course* (2nd ed.) (pp. 305–337). Thousand Oaks, CA: Sage.

Matto, H. C. (2011). Young adulthood. In E. D. Hutchison (Ed.) and Contributors, *Dimensions of human behavior: The changing life course* (4th ed.) (pp. 269–303). Thousand Oaks, CA: Sage.

McCarter, S. A. (2011). Adolescence. In E. D. Hutchison (Ed.) and Contributors, *Dimensions of human behavior: The changing life course* (4th ed.) (pp. 220–268). Thousand Oaks, CA: Sage.

McWhirter, J. J., McWhirter, B. T., McWhirter, E. H., & McWhirter, R. J. (2007). *At risk youth* (4th ed.). Belmont, CA: Brooks/Cole.

Milevsky, A. (2011). *Sibling relationships in childhood and adolescence: Predictors and outcomes*. New York: Columbia University Press.

Muntigl, P. (2004). Ontogenesis in narrative therapy: A linguistic-semiotic examination of client change. *Family Process*, 43(1), 109–131.

Nadeau, R. (2008). Using the visual arts to expand personal creativity. In B. Warren (Ed.), *Using the creative arts in therapy and healthcare* (pp. 43–63). East Sussex, UK: Routledge.

Newman, B. M., & Newman, P. R. (2006). *Development through life: A psychosocial approach* (9th ed). Belmont, CA: Thomson Wadsworth.

Newman, B. M., & Newman, P. R. (2012). *Development through life: A psychosocial approach* (11th ed). Belmont, CA: Wadsworth.

Nichols, M. P., & Schwartz, R. C. (2006). *Family therapy: Concepts and methods* (7th ed). Boston, MA: Pearson.

Phillips, S. D., Burns, B. J., Wagner, H. R., Kramer, T. L., & Robbins, J. M. (2002). Parental incarceration among adolescents receiving mental health services. *Journal of Child and Family Services*, 11(4), 385–399.

Rabin, M. (2003). *Art therapy and eating disorders*. New York: Columbia University Press.

Raley, R. K., Crissey, S., & Muller, C. (2007). Of sex and romance: Late adolescent relationships and young adult union formation. *Journal of Marriage and Family*, 69, 1210–1226. doi: 10.1111/j.1741-3737.2007.00442.x

Raske, M. B. (2005). The disability discrimination model in social work practice. In G. E. May & M. B. Raske (Eds.), *Ending disability discrimination: Strategies for social workers* (pp. 99–112). Boston, MA: Pearson.

Rhodes, J. E., Grossman, J. B., & Resch, N. L. (2000). Agents of change: Pathways through which mentoring relationships influence adolescents' academic adjustment. *Child Development*, 71, 1662–1671. doi: 10.1111/1467-8624.00256

Riley, S. (2003). Using art therapy to address adolescent depression. In C. A. Malchiodi (Ed.), *Handbook of art therapy* (pp. 220–228). New York: The Guilford Press.

Rossi, M. H., & Mackie, K. L. (2011). Feelings landscape. In S. Degges-White & N. L. Davis (Eds.), *Integrating the expressive arts into counseling practice: Theory-based interventions* (pp. 96–97). New York: Springer Publishing Company.

Saleebey, D. (1997). *The strengths perspective in social work practice* (2nd ed.). New York: Longman.

Saleebey, D. (2002). Introduction: Power in the people. In D. Saleebey (Ed.), *The strengths perspective in social work practice* (3rd ed., pp. 1–22). Boston, MA: Allyn & Bacon.

Saleebey, D. (2002). The strengths approach to practice. In D. Saleebey (Ed.), *The strengths perspective in social work practice* (3rd ed., pp. 80–93). Boston, MA: Allyn & Bacon.

Saleebey, D. (2002). *The strengths perspective in social work practice* (3rd ed.). Boston: Allyn & Bacon.

Schulenberg, J., & Maggs, J.L. (1997). *Health risks and developmental transitions during adolescence*. Cambridge, UK: Cambridge University Press.

Seymour, F. W., & Epston, D. (1989). An approach to childhood stealing with evaluation of 45 cases. *Australian & New Zealand Journal of Family Therapy*, 10(3), 137–143.

Shapiro, J., & Ross, V. (2002). Application of narrative theory and therapy to the practice of family medicine. *Family Medicine*, 34(20), 96–100.

Sharry, J., Madden, B., & Darmody, M. (2003). *Becoming a solution detective: Identifying your clients' strengths in practical brief therapy*. Binghamton, NY: The Haworth Clinical Practice Press.

Shriver, S. P., Byer, C. O., Shainberg, L. W., & Galliano, G. (2002). *Dimensions of human sexuality* (6th ed). New York: McGraw-Hill Higher Education.

Sigelman, C. K., & Rider, E. A. (2012). *Life-span human development* (7th ed). Belmont, CA: Wadsworth.

Silver, E., Williams, A., Worthington, F., & Phillips, N. (1998). Family therapy and soiling: An audit of externalizing and other approaches. *Journal of Family Therapy*, 20, 413–422.

Slattery, J. M. (2004). *Counseling diverse clients: Bringing context into therapy*. Belmont, CA: Brooks/Cole.

Slivinske, J., & Slivinske, L. (2011). *Storytelling and other activities for children in therapy*. Hoboken, NJ: John Wiley & Sons.

Stallard, P. (2009). *Anxiety: Cognitive behaviour therapy with children and young people*. London, UK: Routledge.

St-James-O'Connor, T., Meakes, E., Pickering, M., & Schuman, M. (1997). On the right track: Client experience of narrative therapy. *Contemporary Family Therapy: An International Journal*, 19, 479–495.

Thomas, A. J., & Schwarzbaum, S. E. (Eds). (2011). *Culture & identity: Life stories for counselors and therapists* (2nd ed). Thousand Oaks, CA: Sage Publications, Inc.

Tuttle, D., & Tuttle, N. (1996). *Self-esteem and adjusting with blindness: The process of responding to life's demands*. Springfield, IL: Charles C. Thomas.

United Nations. (1948). *United Nations Universal Declaration of Human Rights*. Retrieved September 21, 2011 from http://www.un.org/en/documents/udhr/.

U. S. Department of Veteran Affairs, National Center for PTSD. (2009). *How deployment stress affects children and families: Research findings*. Retrieved May 25, 2011 from www.ptsd.va.gov/professional/pages/pro_deployment_stress_children.asp.

Vromans, L. P., & Schweitzer, R. D. (2011). Narrative therapy for adults with major depressive disorder: Improved symptom and interpersonal outcomes. *Psychotherapy Research*. 21(1), 4–15, doi: 10.1080/10503301003591792.

Wade, A. (1997). Small acts of living: Everyday resistance to violence and other forms of oppression. *Contemporary Family Therapy*, 19(1), 23–39.

Wainright, J. L., Russell, S. T., & Patterson, C. J. (2004). Psychosocial adjustment, school outcomes, and romantic relationships of adolescents with same-sex parents. *Child Development*, 75, 1886–1898. doi: 10.1111/j.1467-8624.2004.00823.x

Walsh, J. (2007). *Endings in clinical practice: Effective closure in diverse settings* (2nd ed). Chicago, IL: Lyceum Books, Inc.

Wang, H., Kao, G., & Joyner, K. (2006). Stability of interracial and intraracial relationships among adolescents. *Social Science Research*, 35(2), 435–453.

Wanner, S. Y. (1994). *On with the story: Adolescents learning through narrative*. Portsmouth, NH: Boynton/Cook Publishers, Inc.

Weber, M., Davis, K., & McPhie, L. (2006). Narrative therapy, eating disorders, and groups: Enhancing outcomes in rural NSW. *Australian Social Work*, 59(4), 391–405. doi: 10.1080/03124070600985970.

Weis, R. (2008). *Introduction to abnormal child and adolescent psychology*. Thousand Oaks, CA: Sage Publications, Inc.

Weston, H. E., Boxer, P., & Heatherington, L. (1998). Children's attributions about family arguments: Implications for family therapy. *Family Process*, 37, 35–49.

White, M. (2004). *Narrative practice and exotic lives: Resurrecting diversity in everyday life*. Adelaide, South Australia: Dulwich Centre Publications.

White, M. (2007). *Maps of narrative practice*. New York: W. W. Norton.

White, M., & Epston, D. (1990). *Narrative means to therapeutic ends*. New York: W. W. Norton.

Worden, J. W. (2009). *Grief counseling and grief therapy: A handbook for the mental health practitioner* (4th ed). New York: Springer Publishing Company, LLC.

Glossary

Adjustment Process to Blindness—Dean and Naomi Tuttle delineate seven phases of adjustment to blindness including physical or social trauma, shock and denial, mourning and withdrawal, succumbing and depression, reassessment and reaffirmation, coping and mobilization, and self-acceptance and self-esteem. Each person may progress through these stages in a unique manner. In a sense, those who lose their vision move through stages similar to the bereaved, except they are mourning the loss of functioning, both social and physical.

Anorexia—A condition characterized by excessive weight loss, refusal of many foods, obsessive exercise, and feeling that one is overweight, even though one is well below a healthy weight.

Anxiety—Feelings of worry and apprehension often accompanied by physiological changes.

Art therapy—A type of therapy in which communication, understanding, insight, and expression of emotions is facilitated through the creation of personalized artwork or creative activity. Many clients may feel safer and less afraid to express themselves when using drawing, painting, or sculpting than when engaged in more traditional types of talk therapies.

Binge eating—A condition characterized by eating extremely large amounts of food.

Bulimia—Those with bulimia tend to binge eat, and then vomit or abuse laxatives to avoid gaining weight.

Community violence—Violence occurring in the context of the neighborhood or community setting.

Co-construction of stories—In the context of therapy, when practitioners and clients tell or write narratives together. Reflection of themes back to clients can be an important component of co-constructing their stories. These reflections can prove interesting to clients and provide the opportunity for the gaining of insight into oneself and life situations.

Co-narration—In the context of therapeutic storytelling, when the therapist assists in the telling of the story with the client.

Controlled breathing—This technique may be modified to suit the preferences and needs of individuals, and it involves slowly breathing deeply, holding the breath, and then slowly releasing the breath.

Coping—Methods that allow individuals positive ways to manage their emotions by using techniques such as journaling, meditating, exercising to relieve stress, sharing emotions with trusted people, and developing problem-solving skills.

Cumulative disadvantage—Those risk-factors that cumulatively place a person in an unfavorable position in life such as having an incarcerated parent, poverty, exposure to substance abuse, and violence.

Dating violence—Dating relationships in which violence can be damaging to an individual's self-esteem at a minimum. It also may be dangerous, resulting in serious injury or death for the victims of dating violence. Violence in dating relationships may take many forms, including verbal and emotional abuse, physical assault, sexual assault, threatening to kill or actually murdering one's partner, harming pets, intimidating behavior, and stalking.

Deconstruction—Breaking down, or deconstructing fictitious or autobiographical stories and then rewriting, or reconstructing them may be a powerful experience contributing to growth, healing, and feelings of control over one's environment and life.

Externalization—In narrative therapy, this involves objectification of a problem. In this fashion, a therapist helps individuals see that they are not the problem, but that the problem in and of itself is the problem. The problem itself becomes a major focus of treatment.

Gradual Self-Disclosure Storytelling Technique—In the context of storytelling, Johanna and Lee Slivinske discuss this method utilizing four distinct levels of inquiry to assist clients who are uncomfortable with self-disclosure. Level-one questions enable clients to simply answer questions regarding characters in the story. It is hoped that clients will identify with characters' situations and gain insight into themselves through this experience. Level-two questions are written in such a manner that individuals may answer questions relating to someone other than themselves, such as a friend or family member, who has had experiences similar to characters in the story. This allows for slightly more disclosure from the client. Level-three questions directly address emotional issues relevant to the client's life, by asking questions specifically posed about how the client's situation is similar to the situation of the story's characters. This level requires even more disclosure about a person's own life. Level-four requires the highest level of disclosure. The individual is asked to finish the ending to his or her own story, by writing about, talking about, or drawing the ending.

Grief—Feelings of extreme sadness and loss, usually related to the death of a loved one. It may also be associated with other losses experienced in life, such as developing a disability.

Guided imagery—A relaxation technique in which a person envisions a comforting or calming setting in his or her mind. It may be an amusement park on a sunny day, a calm and serene lake, the ocean, or any place that provides feelings of positive emotional responses. A person may imagine a particular environment, including sensory experiences pertinent to that environment.

High-risk behaviors—Behaviors involving reckless sexuality, drug and alcohol use, violence, and so forth which may occur in acting-out youth.

Hope—A belief that something positive will occur in the future.

Identity formation—Adolescents and young adults may participate in experimentation with various life roles, which hopefully will contribute to a permanent finding of the self, or the discovery of whom one is.

Identity versus role confusion—When faced with the psychosocial crisis of identity versus role confusion, a part of Erik Erikson's Psychosocial Theory, an adolescent is confronted with establishing a firm identity, or finding out who one truly is. This entails discovering unknown or unexplored aspects of oneself. A person during adolescence often struggles with finding out who he or she is, and how he or she fits into one's society.

Independent living skills—Tasks which must be mastered in order to successfully achieve independence including the ability to earn and manage money and financial responsibilities, the knowledge of how to grocery shop and cook, the maturity and diligence to maintain a decently clean living environment, and the ability to care for one's self, and sometimes others.

Individuation—Adolescents and young adults may struggle with attempts to formulate their own identities. This is a typical and expected part of development, especially within the context of Western cultural expectations, whereas adolescents may distance themselves from parents or caregivers in order to further the development of self. This "breaking away" or individuation may contribute to adolescent and parental conflicts, particularly when teens and parents hold incongruent beliefs and value systems.

Intimacy versus isolation—Young adulthood, according to Erik Erikson's Psychosocial Theory, involves the psychosocial crisis of intimacy versus isolation. During this time period in one's life, an individual struggles to solidify close relationships including but not limited to those with intimate partners, friends and family. One prepares for and possibly becomes firmly rooted in a committed relationship to meet the demands of the challenges of developing intimacy. According to Erikson, if a person successfully builds a close and trusting relationship with another person, then he or she has successfully overcome the psychosocial crisis of intimacy versus isolation. If a person is unable to achieve this, he or she may feel isolated and lonely, lacking close emotional contact in personal relationships.

Lifemapping—Utilizing a visual representation of shapes connected by arrows to draw or write about one's life story.

Love—Feelings of fondness, bonding, and affection between people.

Mutual storytelling technique—Richard Gardner described his technique as a method of communication with children involving active storytelling with a therapist and child client participating. Upon hearing a child's story, the therapist may select important themes, use the same characters, and create a story that has more positive adaptations and outcomes.

Narrative therapy—A therapy method utilizing storytelling and personal recollection as important mechanisms through which a person may express a variety of problems. This method uses therapeutic questioning that would enable clients to identify important issues and assist them in reformulating more positive directions and outcomes to their situations. Therapists may assist clients to deconstruct their stories and by assigning meaning. Externalization or objectification of the problem may also be utilized. Also, therapists may assist clients in retelling their stories.

Peer-group—Teens and young adults often are influenced by their friends and same age classmates, and try to "fit in" with one particular group.

Phototherapy—A creative method of treatment using photos to elucidate cognitions, emotions, and client narratives. Photos serve as springboards for therapeutic conversations, and depict a point of departure to delve deeper into clients' thoughts, feelings, and narratives.

PLAN Method of Intervention—The PLAN method of intervention developed by Johanna and Lee Slivinske provides concrete steps and actions that can be taken to formulate goals, action plans, and build upon strengths. When using the PLAN method, the following steps can be applied to treatment of individuals' personalized challenges and strengths. The PLAN method of intervention for adolescents and young adults involves the following concepts: **P**ositive action creates positive lifestyles. **L**ook to the future. **A**ctivate your strengths, both inside and out. **N**ever give up on yourself.

Positive peer group identity—A concept in which friends and classmates will influence peers to participate in healthy activities such as athletics, academics, clubs, and civic organizations. These friends and activities may serve as buffers against the challenging realities of everyday life. They also may provide enjoyment, the opportunity for recreational activities, and the necessary social connections to meet and develop an intimate relationship.

Possibility questions—Questions that help individuals define who they are and what they desire from their lives. These are especially significant during the teen and young adulthood years, as individuals are in the process of becoming and formulating who they will be, and what they will do, for life.

Post-traumatic stress—People who have experienced traumatic events such as sexual assault or combat may feel afraid, loss of control, helplessness, and terror. This may contribute to symptoms such as flashbacks, nightmares, agitation, detachment, hypervigilance, avoidance, and hopelessness.

Poverty—Living without needed resources and necessities often because of inadequate income. Resources that literally may be lacking from a person's life include basic needs such as clean water, food, clothing, housing, and so forth.

Progressive muscle relaxation—A technique that involves systematically tightening and relaxing various muscle groups, which may provide relief from stress or anxiety.

Progressive storytelling—Another effective method when using storytelling involves use of the progressive story. Using this technique, individuals build upon a story, further developing the plot and adding characters if desired. People may learn vicariously from the experiences of characters in the story.

Psychosocial theory—Erik Erikson developed psychosocial theory, describing eight psychosocial stages and crises that individuals pass through in their lives. When referring to psychosocial crises, he viewed these as typical developmental challenges or conflicts that everyone maneuvers over the life course.

Rape Trauma Syndrome—After a sexual assault, people may exhibit and experience symptoms related to their traumatic experience. Some of these symptoms include: Disorganization Phase: A person feels frightful, angry, and in denial that the rape has occurred. She or he may question how she or he could have avoided the assault, and may blame herself or himself. Controlled Reaction Phase: A person in this phase may appear calmer and less emotional, although she or he is still seriously harmed from the assault. Reorganization Phase: A person adjusts to reintegrating her or his life and adjusting to living from day-to-day after the rape.

Reconstruction—Stories are told and retold, at times with the help of a therapist. By retelling stories with clients, they become empowered and challenged to look toward possibilities in alterations in their thinking and perception, as well as the possibility of positive change. Positive, adaptive, outcomes may be integrated throughout the reconstructed narrative.

Reframing—Through reframing and rewriting stories, individuals have the opportunity for recreating meaning of previous or current life experiences.

Restorying—a. Stories are told and retold, at times with the help of a therapist. By retelling stories with clients, they become empowered and challenged to look toward possibilities in alterations in their thinking and perception, as well as the possibility of positive change. b. In this process, the practitioner borrows another's story, and tells it when it is applicable to another person's life. Through restorying, one may gain insight into self and others, and witness how positive resolutions regarding difficult situations were achieved.

Resilience—Resilience is a term frequently used in the strengths perspective and positive psychology. Resilience focuses on the application of individuals' gifts, assets, and strengths toward the amelioration of challenges and overcoming of obstacles in peoples' lives. Although people may have made less than favorable decisions in the past, in many instances they will actually have ideas or suggestions about what would help them in the future. One way resilience is commonly explained to clients and students is as an ability to "bounce back" from stressful events.

Role-plays—Role-plays may benefit adolescents and young adults in treatment, and stories may be acted out with assistance from a therapist, in a group setting where characters or parts are assigned to individuals, or with family members. Experimentation with new or familiar situations, emotions, and behaviors may occur in this milieu in a relatively safe environment.

Self-care—Taking good care of oneself by partaking in positive activities such as: healthy eating, engaging in exercise, meditating to aid in relaxation and stress relief, writing in a journal, listening to mood enhancing music, using art to express oneself, and so forth.

Self-esteem—The feelings and beliefs, either positive or negative, that one has about oneself.

Sexual abuse—Sexual exploitation of a child or adolescent under the age of 18. This may occur through a variety of means including exposure of genitals to performing sexual acts.

Stages of grief—Elisabeth Kübler-Ross studied the experiences of those living with terminal illnesses. She later formulated five stages that individuals may experience, including denial, anger, bargaining, depression, and acceptance, though not necessarily in a linear form, while experiencing the grieving process.

Story customization—Therapeutic stories may be modified to meet the individualized needs of clients. Practitioners may personalize narratives by changing details of stories, adding clients' names, or altering situations.

Storytelling—A form of narrative often using words and images to tell of what has happened. It is also an important medium for transmitting information, values, and morals from one generation to the next, within the context of immediate and extended familial relationships. Historically speaking, cultural and ethnic traditions and strengths have been passed down in this manner, often involving the oral tradition.

Strengths approach to storytelling—Utilizing positive qualities or strengths including clients' gifts, assets, and abilities to make meaning of stories and experiences, learn lessons, and gain insight.

Strengths-based statements—Affirmative statements or phrases integrated into discussions with clients when appropriate. The statement may then be followed up on by examining how these positive traits, strengths, and relationship assets may be applied to aspects of their personal, academic, and professional lives.

Strengths identification—Searching for and building upon individuals' unique assets and strengths in their lives. Look toward their inner gifts, family supports, friendships (past and present), abilities, desire for change, as well as community-based opportunities and assets. Cultural beliefs, spirituality, and religious values and beliefs can also be built on to solidify a foundation for growth and healthy development.

Strengths perspective—Dennis Saleebey promotes highlighting a client's gifts, assets, and strengths in general. In this approach, practitioners must search for and identify assets, gifts, and positive attributes of clients, families and communities. Strengths include personal and family tales, folklore, and cultural stories.

Strengths-based questions—Questions that promote resilience through facilitating "coping" or "handling" even the most challenging or overwhelming situations. Questions designed to elicit strengths from characters within stories, and from clients.

Therapeutic storytelling—Using stories to help clients to identify strengths and overcome challenges in their own lives.

Author Index

Subject Index

0 1341 1661339 6

Barcode on next page.